Tibetan Buddhist Medicine and Psychiatry

The Diamond Healing

Tibetan Buddhist Medicine and Psychiatry

The Diamond Healing

TERRY CLIFFORD

Foreword by His Holiness the Dalai Lama
Introduction by Lokesh Chandra

Samuel Weiser, Inc.
York Beach, Maine

First published in 1984 by
Samuel Weiser, Inc.
Box 612
York Beach, Maine 03910

First paper edition, 1990

ISBN 0-87728-710-4

Library of Congress Cataloging in Publication Data

Clifford, Terry.
    Tibetan Buddhist medicine and psychiatry.

    Revision of thesis (Ph.D.)—Union Graduate School,
1977.
    Bibliography: p.
    Includes index.
    "Three psychiatric chapters translated from the
Gyu-zhi": p.
    1. Medicine, Tibetan. 2. Medicine, Buddhist.
3. Psychiatry—Tibet (China) I. Title. [DNLM: 1. Medicine, Oriental—China. 2. Religion and psychology.
3. Psychosomatic medicine. WM 61 C638t]
R603.T5C57   1983   616'.00951'5   84-61872

Cover photo is a Thanka of the Medicine Buddha.
From the collection of Stephen King.
© 1990 Stephen King Fisikon
Schwanenhof D-6759 Wolfstein, W. Germany

Printed in the United States of America by
The Maple Vail Book Manufacturing Group

Table of Contents

List of Illustrations

For my parents

THE DALAI LAMA

THEKCHEN CHOELING
McLEOD GANJ 176219
KANGRA DISTRICT
HIMACHAL PRADESH

F O R E W O R D

 Health and happiness are the rights of every individual. That is why it is important to encourage the promotion of different medical systems. While many systems of medicine such as the Tibetan are traditional and ancient, their importance in contributing substantially towards medical sciences particularly in the field of treating psychosomatic and non-infectious diseases should not be ignored.

 I, therefore, welcome this work by Miss Terry Clifford and hope that it will provide the type of information that will assist both medical students and patients in understanding Tibetan medicine better.

December 26, 1981

Preface

This work was undertaken as part of a doctoral program in psychology and religious studies. It was begun simply as an inquiry into the Tibetan medical psychiatric tradition, but expanded to cover Buddhism as medicine and Tibetan medicine in general when it became clear that an understanding of Tibetan psychiatry necessarily includes all these aspects.

In its present form it represents an effort to introduce Tibetan Buddhist medicine and psychiatry within their religious, medical, and historical contexts. As such, it is meant to reflect the unique union of medicine and religion in Buddhism.

The major research was done in 1976 and the writing completed in 1977. This edition includes revisions made in 1980. However, since the subject is so vast, since there is so little published material on it, and since I am not a scholar of the Tibetan language, it will contain some errors and must therefore be considered a work in progress. At the urging of friends interested in the topic and in spite of its deficiencies and imperfections, I am publishing it in this form in the hope that it may generate further interest and research in Tibetan Buddhist medicine, a much neglected and very profound subject. It is my sincere wish that future studies will improve on this present one which is, especially regarding Tibetan psychiatry, in the nature of a pioneer study.

I would like to take this opportunity to express my deepest and heartfelt thanks to my guru, His Holiness Dudjom Rinpoche, for giving his blessings to this project, to His Holiness the 16th Gyalwa Karmapa, for first bestowing the initiation of the Medicine Buddha, and to all the gracious lamas who have taught me the holy Dharma.

Especially I would like to thank Ven. Tulku Pema Wangyal Rinpoche and Prof. Dr. Lokesh Chandra, M.P., without whose support and encouragement, at the end and beginning respectively, this book would never have come into being, and the following people, all of whom helped in the research, explication, and finalization of the work: Ven. Khyentse Rinpoche, Ven. Dodrup Chen Rinpoche, Ven. Thinley Norbu Rinpoche, Ven. Doboom Tulku Rinpoche, Ven. Ngo-Shul Khen Rinpoche, Ven. Khenpo Palden Sherab, Ven. Yeshe Dorje Rinpoche, Ven. Lama Dodrag Amchi, Ven. Amchi Lama Wangla, Ven. Geshe Jamspal, Ven. Lama Sonam Topgyal, Ven. Lama Namdrol Gyatso, Ven. Lodro Thaye, Anila Yangchen-la and her sister Choskyi-la, Dr. Ama Lobsang, Dr. Pema Dorje, E. Gene Smith, Gyurmed Dorje, John Canti, M.B., B. Chir., Dr. Vaidya Bhagwan Dash, Jigme Tsarong, Philip Romero, M.D., Glenn H. Mullin, Jared Rhoton, Ph.D., Arthur Mandelbaum, Bettyann Lopate, Daniel Goleman, Ph.D., Jonathan Kane, M.D., Edwin Bokert, Ph.D., Mary Newman, Ph.D., Edward Henning, Rick Fields, Jim Battaglino, and many friends at Chanteloube. Finally, my thanks go to Donald Weiser and to everyone who crafted the manuscript into a book.

Terry Clifford

Introduction

by

Dr. Lokesh Chandra*

Ever since Terry Clifford walked into my study to look through nerved xylographs in Tibetan and to consult works on Tibetan medicine in English, some of them going back to 1835 and as rare as stars in the day, she has impressed me by her dedication. Her resolve to understand the uncharted riches of Tibet's medical lore, and her hard work over the years has borne fruit in the present book—a lucid exposition of the subject which is so fluent, so simple, that Tibetan medicine can become the property of every person.

She has specifically chosen to translate the psychiatric chapters of the *Four Tantras* or *Gyu-zhi* to widen our perceptions from ethnopsychiatry, and has tried to correlate the Tibetan expressions with modern psychiatric disturbances. In her concluding remarks she rightly suggests, "So may the inspiration and insight of Tibetan medicine find new expression in yet unimagined ways."

The Diamond Healing will usher in a new understanding of Indo-Tibetan medicine. It summons its intrepid readers to explore further shores of this transcendent system, which is a holistic approach viewing the individual as a healthy being in body and mind while disease indicates a disturbance of this homeostasis. Tibetan medicine treats the individual as a whole in which the physical and trans-

*Director, International Academy of Indian Culture, New Delhi; author and editor of three hundred books published to preserve the wisdom of classical Asia, including the *Tibetan-Sanskrit Dictionary*, *Materials for a History of Tibetan Literature*, *Studies in Indo-Asian Art & Culture*, works on the materia medica of Tibet, *The Classic of Eighteen Topics*, *A New Tibeto-Mongol Pantheon*, *The Mongolian Kanjur* (vols. 1-108).

physical faculties combat the disequilibrium of his total being. Contemporary science has gone a long way to establish that the universe is non-material, matter is energy, space is real and processes are as valid as facts, and that the principle of complementarity validates the subjective content of human experience. *The Diamond Healing* illuminates the living order of Tibetan wisdom to bring a universal frame of reference to replace the broken image of mechanical notions of the 19th century.

Tibetan medicine is a confluent trinity of the Indic, Hellenic and Sinic traditions of medicine wherein the spatial tangents have met and harmonized. The Buddhist *oikumene* provides Tibetan medicine a cosmo-the-andric vision in which the center is neither in the cosmos, nor in the divine (theos), nor in man (andros). It is a center to be found in the intersection of the three. Terry Clifford seeks to inject a transcreative trinity of time into the study of Tibetan medicine, interpreting the legacy of the past in the language of today to give birth to new qualitative parameters for medical science in the future.

The medical lore of Tibet is primarily based on the Ayurveda of India. Seventeen Sanskrit texts were translated into Tibetan and they cover six huge tomes of the Tanjur, the collection of Tibetan canonical classics which have enjoyed the devotion of the pious and the dedication of learned minds of the Land of Snows for a millenium. In all they contain over four thousand imposing pages of classical learning that await adventurous minds ready to explore their riches.

The earliest Indian medical text to be rendered into Tibetan seems to be the *Gyu-zhi* or *Four Tantras* by Chandranandana. Translated in the eighth century, it has been the fundamental classic ever since, used in medical practice and commented upon century after century. The Regent of the Fifth Dalai Lama, Sangye Gyatso, wrote an extensive commentary on this text in the 17th century which has overshadowed all its predecessors in its comprehensiveness and clarity of understanding.

The most prolific translator of Indic texts on medicine was the untiring Rinchen Zangpo who lived from 958 to 1055 A.D. In collaboration with Jalandhara of India, he translated the *Ashtanga-hridaya* of Vagbhata and its commentary by Chandranandana. He was also responsible for the Tibetan translation of a veritable encyclopedia of veterinary science: the principles of horse medicine (hippiatry).

In the 13th century Ratnashri (1228-1308 A.D.) translated Sanskrit texts on alchemy into Tibetan with the help of a yogin and scholars. The original Sanskrit texts are lost, and their Tibetan versions are unique works on tonic elixirs of broad spectrum used to restore the organism to health.

Dharmapala, the great translator of Zhalu, is well known as the systematizer of grammatical literature in Tibet. He lived from 1441 to 1528 A.D. He translated the *Treasury of Roots,* a compendium of grand remedies by the famous Nagarjuna. It is a formulary of roots (accompanied by mantras) for the treatment of nervous and cutaneous disorders, fevers, eye and other diseases. It is also a precious work on psychosomatic treatments.

The great Fifth Dalai Lama, Lobsang Gyatso (1617-1682 A.D.) was the most outstanding statesman and foremost writer of Tibet. He enriched his country with historical works, liturgical treatises, handbooks on propitiatory methods of various deities, compendious works on metaphysics, subtle commentaries on the summa of Buddhism, works on metrics, rhetorics, literary criticism, stylistics, and medicine. He embellished his land with temples and monasteries with funds flowing from the zeal and piety of the Mongolian nobles who flocked to Lhasa loaded with gifts. The Fifth Dalai Lama renewed the tradition of inviting Indian pandits to Tibet, and they inspired fresh interest in the translation of secular disciplines such as the medical sciences.

The court physician of the Fifth Dalai Lama, Dharmo Manrampa, had the biography of the famous Tibetan doctors Yuthog Senior and Junior engraved on woodblocks for printing. He, along with others, commissioned the translation of new Sanskrit medical texts into Tibetan from Hdar. They collated extracts from the works of ten celebrated physicians of India on etiology, hygiene, opium and alum therapy, medico-tantric formulas, series of magic diagrams, and diverse pathologic considerations; it is a sprawling amalgam of disparate components based on practical experience which was completed at the Potala Palace in 1644 A.D. Their second work is on the methods of treatment of Doctor Danadasa; it is accompanied by seventy-two esoteric medical chakras. The third treatise, a medico-alchemical compilation done with the assistance of Doctor Raghunatha from Mathura (near Delhi), includes procedures for the preparation of metallic remedies. It was followed by a collection of occult remedies for maladies produced by *pishaca* and *graha,** transmitted by the physician Raghunatha to the great Lotsava

---

*Types of demonic forces that cause disease.

Lhundup. The last work to be included into the Tibetan canon of the Tanjur was a practical memorandum on hygiene, therapeutics and surgery for eye diseases entitled *Regenerator of Vision.*

Four works of Nagarjuna were rendered into Tibetan, including the *Yoga Shataka* and *Jiva Sutra.* The *Yoga Shataka* was one of the most popular books of medical prescriptions. It was in use from Central Asia to Sri Lanka. Its three folios have been recovered from Central Asia in the local Kuchean language, which is cognate to European languages. The book was translated into Kuchean around 650 A.D. The *Siddha Sara* of Ravigupta was also done into Tibetan. It was a widely popular treatise. Fragments of its Uigur Turkish translation have even been unearthed from the sands of Central Asia.

The transference of medical sciences from India to Tibet was a continuous tradition over a millenium beginning in the eighth century and fostered until the 17th century. These translations were assimilated by Tibetan scholars and furthered through commentaries and practical handbooks. Personal memoranda of a few folios covering the most used prescriptions were written down by eminent doctors and were xylographed for daily use.

Tibetan medicine gained new strength by assimilating the Greek system via Persia. Chinese medicine and materia medica added another dimension to Tibet's medical lore. From the inception it underwent modulations and harmonizations based on experience modified by the alpine context. It was a continuing search for authenticity and equilibrium in man's body, characterized by the deepest in man and nature from the perception of Buddhist serenity.

The medical sciences of Tibet are a continuation and amplification of those of India. Thus they are the culmination of five millenia of man's way to the threshold of a wholesome life of harmonized existence, of his experience of a full sentience. Excavations on ancient India sites of the third millenium B.C. have brought to light several substances like the *shilajatu* (a remedy for diabetes, rheumatism, etc.), leaves of the tree *Azadirachta indica,* horns of the red deer, and skulls on which cranial surgery had been performed—all of which point to the great antiquity of the medical sciences in India. In the Vedic period, which has been dated from 5000 B.C. to 2000 B.C., medicine was already an established profession. *Rig Veda* 9.112 speaks of the healing of fractures and 10.97 is dedicated to healing herbs. The Ashvins were famed physicians and wonder-working surgeons, adepts in treating blindness, paralysis, and rejuvenation; they replaced the lost leg of a soldier with an iron one. The *Atharva Veda,* which is considered to be the source of all Ayurveda or the classical medicine of India, speaks of the use of a unidentified plant, *kushtha,* to combat malarial fever. It speaks of prosthetic limbs, artificial eyes and newly set dentures!

During the lifetime of the Buddha lived Jivaka, the "thrice crowned king" of physician-surgeons. He was an expert in pediatrics and even excelled in brain surgery. He successfully performed intricate abdominal operations. He was a disciple of the renowned Atreya of Taxila, a pioneer in India's history of the medical sciences. During his reign, Emperor Ashoka provided hospitals throughout his dominions and even beyond in the lands on its frontier, "...and as far as Sri Lanka and of the Greek King named Antiochus...medicinal herbs whether useful to man or to beast, have been brought and planted wherever they did not grow." Megastehenes, the Greek ambassador to the court of the Maurya Emperor (third century, B.C.), recorded the high level of India's attainments in obstetrics, preventive medicine and dietetics. Medical science continued to find ever widening avenues of development in India over the centuries.

Tibetan fastness, untouched by war, preserved the rich heritage of Indian medicine until the Chinese occupation. The Chakpori Medical College at Lhasa was the oldest institution of its kind. Indo-Tibetan medicine traveled to the Khalkhas, Inner Mongols and the distant Buryats of northeast Siberia. Here I recall my meeting with Dr. P. Cyrill von Korvin-Krasinski who had specialized in Siberian medicine. When I met him in Germany, he related how he had the privilege of having W. Badmayev as his guru in Mongolian Ayurveda in Warsaw. Badmayev was from the family of Mongolian lama-doctors, one of whom had become court physician to Czar Alexander II. His cousin was the Siberian doctor N.N. Badmayev, who was well known in Leningrad for his Ayurvedic practice and his great success in this therapy. His patients included prominent people like author Alexi Tolstoy, communist leaders such as Bukharin and Rydov, and on some occasions he was even summoned to visit Stalin. The People's Commissar of Health, Kaminsky, had such a high opinion of him that a special Ayurvedic department was established under Dr. Feodorov at Leningrad. Even Professor Ilin of the Military Medical Academy was in this department. During a purge, the department was abolished and the persons liquidated. However, W. Badmayev had fled to Poland where Dr. Krasinski met him. Dr. Krasinski related that Badmayev had given him a number of Siberian medical preparations. I requested him to show me one. He brought a bottle and spoke about its efficacy and was very sad that now he would not have it again, as his guru Badmayev was no longer alive. I requested that Dr. Krasinski show me a bit of his admirable drug. And lo! it was the ubiquitous *hingvashtaka churna,** found in every household of Tibet and India. The splendour of Indo-Tibetan medicine seeks new growth from its silent vastness.

Terry Clifford's effort to unravel Tibetan medicine tempts us to view the wholeness of man and the wedding of the world's civilizations as we seek solutions to the problem of suffering in a convergence of humanistic, spiritual and scientific man becoming one.

---

*An Ayurvedic medicinal formula of eight ingredients, the main one being *ferula assafoetida.*

Part I

Tibetan Buddhist Medicine

NAMO MAHA BHAIKANZEYA

Honour to the Great Medical Buddha!

Whoever due to wrong ideas and attitudes
Is bound to fall into states of suffering,
If he even hears the sound of your sacred name,
He will not be reborn in sorrow
And will reach the state of immaculate purity.

—from Chagmed Rinpoche's
Hymn in Praise of the Medical Buddha

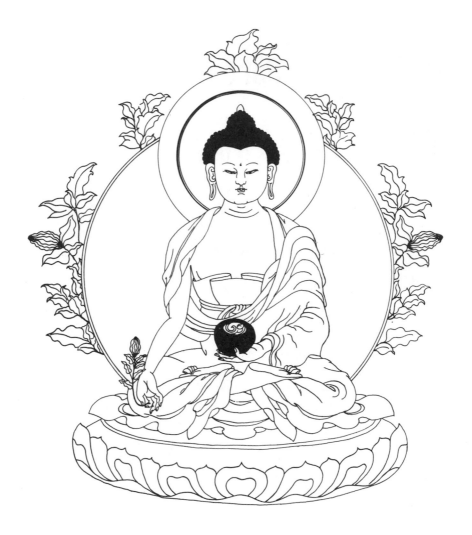

Figure 1 The Medicine Buddha, the Teacher of Medicine: the King of Lapis Lazuli Light (Bhaishajyaguru, Sangye Menla, Vaidurya). His radiant body is azure blue; in his lap he holds a begging bowl full of long-life nectar. As a sign that he gives protection from illness, his right hand is outstretched in the gesture of giving and holds the "great medicine," the myrobalan plant (a-ru-ra).

1

An Overview

Tibetan medicine is a unique system of healing and one of the world's oldest surviving medical traditions. Yet Tibetan Buddhist medicine has been largely ignored by Western scholars and has still to take its rightful place in the history of medicine as known in the West. This work is an attempt to present a general picture of Tibetan Buddhist medicine—its philosophy and history, its cosmology and deities, its treatments and ethics—and to give an in-depth look at its psychiatric tradition, which is, in fact, the world's oldest surviving complete and written system of medical psychiatry.

The medical tradition of Tibet was imported with Buddhism from India in approximately the seventh century A.D. At that time, Indian Ayurvedic medicine was at its height. It had developed for 1,000 years as a highly advanced and written tradition and had even earlier oral antecedents reaching back to Vedic times.

In the centuries that followed the exportation of classical Ayurveda to Tibet, the Indian medical tradition was broken and in part lost in its native land. However, it was preserved in Tibet, where it was further enriched with Chinese and Persian contributions. The Tibetans joined all this to their pre-Buddhist shamanic traditions and have continued to enlarge and develop their medical system up until the present day.

The medicine of Tibet is unique for its blend of spiritual, "magical" and rational healing practices. The remarkable effectiveness of Tibetan medicine was renowned throughout Central Asia, and

Tibet came to be known as the "country of medicine" and the "land of medicine plants." Today, however, this ancient system of healing is in danger of being lost forever.

Tibetan Buddhist medicine is now a system in exile, struggling for existence like the rest of classical Tibetan culture. This situation is due to historical circumstances, to the fact that Chinese communism has forcibly displaced Tibetan Buddhism as the exclusive and dominant factor in all aspects of Tibetan life. When the Chinese took over Tibet in 1959, one hundred thousand Tibetans went into exile, among them many of the great Tibetan lamas but few of the great Tibetan doctors. They are the last generation from the thousand-year-

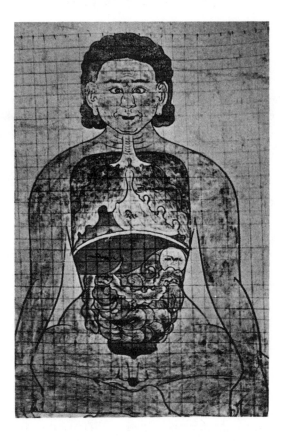

Figure 2 Tibetan anatomical chart showing the internal organs labeled with their names in Tibetan script. The grid represents a basic scale of measurement which is adjusted to individual body size. For example, the length of the thumb equals two units, as seen here.

old culture of Buddhist Tibet and the first Tibetan generation to come in widespread contact with the modern world.

In order to preserve the medical tradition in exile, a small Tibetan Medical Centre with a dispensary, clinic, hospital and medical school has been established in Dharamsala, India, by His Holiness the Dalai Lama. It serves the medical needs of the refugee community and has expanded to out-patient departments in Tibetan settlements throughout the sub-continent.[1] In addition, there are a number of independent and unaffiliated Tibetan doctors and lama-doctors who continue to practice their ancient art in India and the Himalayan countries.

It has been reported that in contemporary Tibet the Chinese, with their great respect for medicine, have preserved much of the medical tradition of that land, particularly the vast array of traditional Tibetan herbal treatments (which are now exported to virtually all provinces of China). But to whatever extent the Chinese may have preserved the Tibetan medical tradition, we can presume that they have removed the religious and spiritual aspects that are not only part and parcel of the whole system but its very source and foundation.

It is precisely this spiritual and philosophical core that makes Tibetan medicine so unique. Indeed, there is no other medical tradition in the world that is so coherently developed in terms of a philosophy and metaphysics. The relationship between Buddhism and healing is innate and extraordinary.

To understand this basic relationship, one need only recognize that the Buddha himself spoke of ultimate truth in terms of a medical analogy. It has been said that the entire teaching of the Buddha is how to prevent suffering. According to the Buddha, we suffer from the inherent frustration of conditioned existence, and our suffering is caused by the fact of impermanence of all entities and by the endless craving that arises from the basic delusion of ego's self-existence. The medicine the Buddha prescribed to overcome our suffering and delusion is his teaching, the Dharma. And the essence of this teaching is to tame the mind and transmute the negative emotions. The Buddha taught that mind is the basis of all phenomena. Mind creates matter and mind creates illness and wellness. And herein lies the fundamental psychosomatic assumption of Buddhist medicine.

Buddhism is primarily a psychological religion, as opposed to a theological one. It aims at understanding the nature of mind and at developing awareness and compassion. The practice of the Buddha's medicine of Dharma relies on one's own efforts, on the recognition of impermanence, on the control of mind, and on the diminishing of craving.

From the Buddhist point of view, physical illness and suffering can be a support to deepen the aspiration towards enlightenment. It can also be used to help us develop compassion. While we are sick, we can turn our suffering into the path. Through the practice of Dharma we can recognize the negative habits and patterns that create suffering and disease and can diminish them.

Buddhism's psychological tenets are set forth in the section of scriptures called Abhidharma. This literature provides the philosophical basis of Buddhist psychology and includes an exacting analysis and classification of the nature of consciousness and mental functioning.

According to the Buddha and Abhidharma, what obscures or prevents the perfection of the human mind are the *klesha* (Sanskrit; Tibetan: *nyon-mongs*). In English they are called afflictive emotions, defilements, mental distortions, negative emotions or even disturbing concepts. In the *Abhidharmasamuccaya* a klesha is defined as a "mental factor that, upon occurring in the mind, has the function of producing turmoil in and lack of control over the psyche."[2] These mental-emotional obscurations are reflexive modes of consciousness, habitual reactive and emotive complexes; they are the psychic roots of illness.

All the thousands of kleshas can be condensed into the so-called "three poisons"—confusion, attachment and aversion, which all arise from fundamental ignorance or unawareness. Obscurations are also classified into two basic groups and sub-groups: 1. emotional patterns, a) gross—acquired in this life, b) subtle—inborn; 2. mental obscurations, a) gross—wrong views, b) subtle—subject-object dualism. It is this latter group, subject-object dualism or holding to the idea of a permanent separate "self," which is the fundamental ignorance that gives rise to all the others. According to Buddhist philosophy, psychology and medicine, this ego-clinging is the source of all delusion, suffering and disease. As it says very clearly in the major Tibetan medical work:

> There is but one cause for all illness, and this is ignorance due to not understanding the meaning of identitylessness [lack of a permanent ego]. For example, even when a bird soars in the sky, it does not part from its shadow. (Likewise,) even when all creatures live and act with joy, because they have ignorance, it is impossible for them to be free of illness.[3]

Tibetan Buddhist medicine is a fascinating and complex interweaving of religion, mysticism, psychology, and rational medicine. It includes a whole array of ideas and concepts that are used for healing along with actual medicaments and treatments. Ultimately, however, it is the product of an ancient culture very different from our own. To the modern person first encountering the Tibetan system of healing, particularly its psychiatric tradition, it may seem alien and remote, archaic and even incomprehensible, especially to a person unacquainted with Buddhism, with which it is so inseparably linked. It is difficult to bridge the gap between a world view of a millennium old sacred culture and that of the scientific materialism of modern times, especially from a medical point of view, yet it is not impossible and not without value.

The study of Tibetan Buddhist medicine, it seems to me, offers a fertile source of information and insight in two ways. First, the tradition's vast body of medical literature, its enormous pharmacopoeia, its unusual methods of diagnosis and treatment, its ethical principles and its philosophic and psychological underpinning are worthy of study, documentation, and preservation per se. They contribute to the history of medicine, medical anthropology and ethnopsychiatry; furthermore, Tibetan medicine's practicability may provide modern medicine with significant contributions.

Secondly, from a theoretical point of view Tibetan medicine offers highly defined and relevant models with which we can enrich our modern views of healing. These include a model of holistic medicine, a model of psychosomatic medicine, a model of mental and psychic healing, an ethical model of the healer, and a model for using illness to develop wisdom.

Tibetan medicine is preeminently holistic. It emphasizes the relationship of mind to body and of the embodied psycho-organism to the universe at large; it makes preventative and curative efforts to maintain and restore cosmic equilibrium within and without. Like most of the world's traditional medical systems, it defines health in terms of balance, but in Tibetan medicine that concept of balance is developed to its furthest and most subtle reaches.

On a relative plane, illness is said to be caused by a lack of harmony within the microcosm or between it and the universe; this includes all the short term causes of disease. But on the absolute plane, illness is understood to be caused by the disharmony originating from the fundamental delusion of duality and ego's self-existence. So while the relative goal of Tibetan medicine is to prevent and cure illness, its ultimate goal is the final cure of all suffering: enlightenment.

Since body and mind are seen as a composite whole, all manner of diagnosis and treatment takes this into account. On the most physical, organic level, the body is understood in terms of humoral theory. The three humors are air, bile, and phlegm. The three humoral constituents of the body are understood to have evolved from the three primary faults or obscurations of mind: phlegm from ignorance, air from craving, and bile from hatred. On the physical plane it is the balance or imbalance of these which is responsible for health and disease.

These humors, it is said, can be influenced by all sorts of natural factors like diet and seasonal changes. They are also said to be influenced by life activities, psychological conditions, astrological and "unseen forces," and finally by spiritual conditions, karma, existing from the present or previous lives.

The concepts of karma and reincarnation are central to Buddhism and Buddhist medicine. Karma can be understood simply as the working out of the law of cause and effect. Every activity of body, speech, and mind, conscious and unconscious, is believed to create its inevitable result in this life or in future lives. In terms of reincarnation, the karmic force that finds itself reborn is not a separate ego-unit or an independent identity. Rather, it is the psycho-moral continuity generated by an individual in past lives, and this karma works itself out with relentless justice as a subtle natural law over successive rebirths.

Since the effects of the karma of previous lives may be felt in the present, some diseases are said to have a purely spiritual or karmic cause. According to Tibetan medicine, these diseases will not respond to ordinary medical treatments, but demand, instead, spiritual or religious treatments to cure them on a level that parallels their source.

The idea of karma and karmic disease is a distinguishing feature of Tibetan Buddhist medicine. Even in the relationship between patient and physician karma can play an important part since, according to the Tibetans, if there is no karmic connection between them, not even the best physician and the most willing patient will be able to effect a cure.

For purposes of study and clarification, I have divided Tibetan medicine into three main categories: Dharmic or religious medicine; tantric or yogic medicine; and somatic or regular medicine. In actual practice these three are integrated.

Dharmic medicine heals through spiritual and psychological practices for realizing the nature of mind and controlling the negative emotions. It includes meditation, moral development, prayer, and other religious practices.

Tantric medicine covers an intermediate level between the mental and the physical. It uses psycho-physical yogic practices to transform subtle vital energies within the body as a means of healing oneself and others. And it often produces psychic or "magical" powers.

From the spiritual and yogic categories of Tibetan medicine come specific religious, meditation and visualization practices for healing. As modern medicine discovers more about the psychosomatic origins of disease, about the affects of the negative emotions on body chemistry, and about the role of faith or positive emotions in the working of the placebo effect, the spiritual, psychic and yogic healing techniques from Tibetan medicine may deepen our insights into the mysterious relationship of mind to healing.

The third category is somatic or regular medicine, which is based on the Indian Ayurvedic system but includes some other foreign and Tibetan contributions. Cures range from a "gentle" system of naturopathy—mineral baths, massage, dietary and environmental adjustments, etc.—to the use of medicines compounded from an extensive herbal pharmacology, as well as acupuncture, cupping, etc.

In all kinds of Tibetan medicine the interactive role of the healer is emphasized. "Affectionate care" is considered to be an important factor in the recovery of the patient. The moral quality of the healer, his or her depth of wisdom and compassion, is believed to be directly related to ability to effect a cure.

The category of somatic or regular Tibetan medicine classically contains eight branches, one of which is psychiatry. Experts in the history of psychiatry have identified three basic and separate trends in the treatment of mental illness: the magico-religious approach; the organic-physical approach; and the psychological-emotional approach.[4] The interesting thing about Tibetan medical psychiatry is that it combines all three.

Unlike modern views of psychosis, which tend to dwell on one approach to the exclusion of all others, i.e. biochemical or psychological, Tibetan psychiatry provides a holistic, albeit unusual, model of the causes and treatment of serious mental disorders.

Five primary causes of insanity are specified: (1) karma; (2) humoral imbalance; (3) poison; (4) emotional factors; (5) unseen negative forces or "demons." Besides karma, the inclusion of demonic forces is, of course, entirely outside the limits of modern psychiatry, and just how these "demons" may be interpreted will be taken up in a later chapter. Suffice it to mention here that the exacting Tibetan identification of symptoms associated with possession by various demons provides a unique system of classification of psychopathology, and one that is not without remarkable parallels in the contemporary scientific classification of mental disorders.

The Tibetans have developed a wide field of psychopharmacology and have an enormous number of psychiatric medicines, none of which have been previously identified or scientifically tested in the West. These psychiatric medicines enjoyed a great reputation for clinical effectiveness in Asia. I personally first heard of them from a usually serene friend who, following a head injury, was given over to unpredictable emotional fits and rages during her convalescence. The Tibetan doctor treating her administered a herbal incense,* a favored Tibetan form of psychiatric medicine, which she reported calmed her down immediately upon inhaling it. And Theodore Burang, who is, to my knowledge, the only Westerner to have examined the whole range of Tibetan psychiatric treatment first-hand in Tibet (in the earlier part of this century), wrote that "the success rate of Tibetan methods in the treatment of mental illness is remarkable."[5]

Since this work deals specifically with documenting the Tibetan psychiatric tradition, I have tried to identify the main substances used in psychiatric medicine. Someday, perhaps, modern scientists may make a thorough examination of Tibetan psychiatric medicines in their laboratories and in clinical trials. After all, the initial breakthrough in contemporary psychopharmacology, the development of the first major tranquilizer, came from scientific research on *Rawolfia serpentina,* a plant used for centuries in India to treat madness.

In order to present authentic textual evidence of the Tibetan psychiatric system, I have included an original translation of three psychiatric chapters from the *Gyu-zhi (rGyud-bzhi)* or *The Four Tantras,* the most famous and fundamental work in Tibetan medical literature. The *Gyu-zhi* is said to contain, in condensed essence form, the entire teaching of Tibetan medicine. This work, whose origin is ascribed to the Medicine Buddha himself, was brought to Tibet from India in the eighth century and was added to over successive centuries. These

---

*It was smoke from smoldering chips of black aloeswood (*ar-ga-ru*).

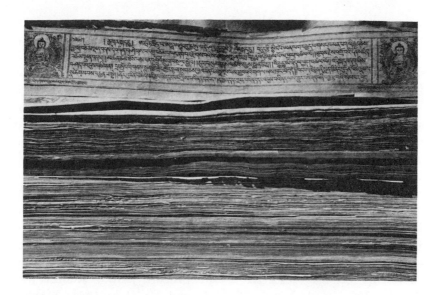

Figure 3 The *Gyu-zhi*, the most important text of Tibetan medicine. This ancient copy was printed from hand-carved blocks and shows Shakyamuni Buddha and the Medicine Buddha on its opening page. Like most Tibetan books, it consists of long, narrow, unbound folios. It was carried out of Tibet by refugees. In contemporary Tibet, most of the irreplaceable treasure of sacred literature has been destroyed by the Chinese, but there is some reason to hope that works on medicine have been preserved.

three chapters from the *Gyu-zhi* represent the oldest psychiatric text in the world still forming the basis for clinical practice.

The entire *Gyu-zhi* has not yet been translated into English. Parts of the Second and Fourth Tantras were translated by Rechung Rinpoche in his book *Tibetan Medicine,* which also contains a concise history of Tibetan medicine and a translation of the biography of Yuthog, the famous Tibetan physician-saint. A full translation of the First Tantra and sections of the Second Tantra of the *Gyu-zhi,* annotated by Dr. Yeshi Dhonden, personal physician to His Holiness the Dalai Lama, has been published by the Library of Tibetan Works and Archives under the title *The Ambrosia Heart Tantra, Vol. I,* and a translation of the rest of the *Gyu-zhi* is now underway there. A recent work by German physician Elisabeth Finckh presents a translation of parts of the *Gyu-zhi*'s First Tantra, details its medical terminology and outlines the whole work.[6] Apart from this, the only other work in English on the *Gyu-zhi* was done by the pioneering Hungarian scholar

Csoma de Koros, who published a complete outline of its chapters in the *Journal of the Asiatic Society of Bengal* in 1835.

There is an enormous body of Tibetan medical literature, but at the time of this writing only one of these books exists in translation. It is a work of Nagarjuna's translated by Dr. Vaidya Bhagwan Dash in his book *Tibetan Medicine: With Special Reference to Yoga Sataka.*[7] The available literature on Tibetan medicine is dismally lacking.[8] There are only a few other modern works in English that deal with the subject: *An Introduction to Tibetan Medicine,* a collection of essays published by the Tibetan Review in India; Burang's *The Tibetan Art of Healing,* which contains a discussion of Tibetan psychiatry; and various essays in Tibet-oriented publications. More generally, Raoul Birnbaum's *The Healing Buddha* discusses the importance of healing in Buddhism, but mainly in reference to Chinese Buddhist scriptures.

The material on Tibetan psychiatry I have presented here represents original research drawn primarily from studies with Tibetan lamas and doctors in India and Nepal in 1976. Material related to Buddhism and Tibetan medicine in general has also been gathered from Tibetan lamas as well as from published sources— especially, regarding medicine, Rechung Rinpoche's seminal work.

Although the Mahayana and Vajrayana Buddhism that was imported to Tibet differs considerably from the early schools of Buddhism in India, and although Buddhism and Buddhist medicine took on in Tibet a distinct flavor and form from that shamanistic land, the wisdom-ground of Tibetan Buddhist medicine originates from the Buddha and his teachings. So let us begin this study of the Tibetan art of healing with the Venerable One and his medicine, the Dharma.

2

The Medicine of Dharma

In Mahayana and Vajrayana Buddhism, which are the schools of Buddhism that were established in Tibet, the concept of Buddhahood goes beyond the figure of the historical Buddha Shakyamuni who lived in India more than two and a half millennia ago.

In the Mahayana and Vajrayana view, Buddhahood is an immanent quality of mind, inherent in all sentient beings whether insects or aristocrats. The purpose of human life, therefore, is to uncover and realize this quality of enlightenment.

According to the Mahayana and Vajrayana, the Primordial Buddha is said to have always existed, yet to transcend the duality of existence or non-existence. From the abiding primordial Buddha-nature, infinite Buddhas have arisen in countless forms in countless epochs and in countless world systems, and they will continue to do so.

Nevertheless, the historical figure of Gautama Buddha or Shakyamuni Buddha is understood as the Buddha who arose for our age and universe. He is the fourth Buddha in a line of a thousand Buddhas who will appear in our universe. The first Buddha was Dipankara, and the next or coming Buddha is Maitreya, the "Buddha of Love." From the Mahayana and Vajrayana point of view, the Buddha was already enlightened when he entered the womb of his mother. But in order to set an example of the path to enlightenment, he went through progressive stages to gain Buddhahood in his own human lifetime and in order to expound his teachings.

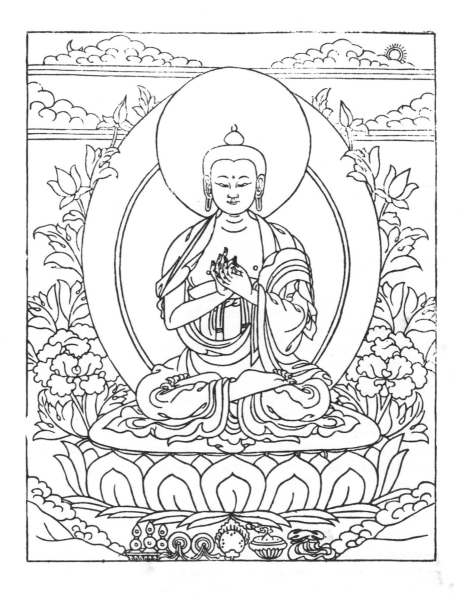

Figure 4 Shakyamuni Buddha, the Great Physician, seated on a lotus throne representing the purity of the wisdom nature within. From the enlightened mind arise countless wisdom activities, one of which is the compassionate science of healing.

Furthermore, as part of his example, the previous lives of the Buddha, his many incarnations during his long career as a bodhisattva, were known to him and are recorded in the Buddhist literature called the *Jataka Tales*. Among his past lives are many incarnations as animals, and this serves to emphasize the sacredness with which all sentient life is held in Buddhism; the Buddha also had past lives as a doctor or healer. During his successive incarnations he developed wisdom and compassion to such an extent that when he took his final rebirth as Prince Gautama, he achieved nirvana and complete Buddhahood and thus passed beyond the realms of birth and death.

Shakyamuni Buddha

He who was to become the Buddha, the "Fully Awakened One," was born Gautama, Prince of the Shakya clan, in Northern India, now Nepal, during the sixth century B.C. His father deliberately protected him from a knowledge of the horrors and difficulties of life, and for twenty-eight years the Prince Gautama lived a life of royal ease and refined sensuality. But going one day beyond the palace gates, he came upon the signs of truth—a sick person, a feeble old man, a corpse and an ascetic. Then he realized that humanity was mired in suffering. Feeling renunciation deep in his heart and leaving behind a life of pleasure and worldly greatness, he fled the palace by night and set off to find the cure for suffering.

Seven years later, after six years of practices of severe austerities that he ultimately dismissed as extremist, he sat absorbed in profound meditation beneath the Bodhi Tree. Throughout a night of assault by the forces of death and desire he remained immovable in meditation, and with the break of dawn, having overcome all the negative forces of mind and life, the Prince became the Buddha, the "Conqueror."

Because of his enormous compassion, a quality that became his hallmark, he taught others the truth that he had, by himself and within himself, discovered as the way out of suffering. His doctrine is called the Dharma.

In his very first teaching the Buddha propounded the doctrine of "The Four Noble Truths." The first truth, he said, is the truth of suffering—existence is painful; the second is the truth of the cause of suffering—selfish craving; the third is the truth of the end of suffering—nirvana, literally "blown out," the complete removal of craving; and the fourth truth is the truth of the path to the end of suffering—the eightfold path summarized as the threefold development of morality, meditation and wisdom.

From the five monks who listened to this first discourse of the Venerable One, there grew up a community of monks, nuns and laity who were the followers of the Buddha and his Dharma. They are called the Sangha, and they represent the living expression of the aspiration to enlightenment. The Buddha, the Dharma, and the Sangha together form the inseparable Buddhist trinity known as "The Three Jewels." The path of the Buddha is also called "The Middle Way" because it relies neither on extreme asceticism nor on sensual indulgence.

For forty-five years the Venerable One gave himself to the training of humanity in the way of the truth for the sake of all sentient beings, emphasizing always the selfless love and goodwill that are both the path and expression of that truth. In his eightieth year, surrounded by his beloved disciples, he passed beyond his body and entered the final Parinirvana. In his last teaching he reiterated the sense of self-responsibility and the recognition of impermanence that are at the heart of Dharma. Comforting and exhorting his mourning disciples, he said: "Everything that is compounded must decay. Be lamps unto yourselves, O monks."

Thus the Buddha, most rare and gentle human, he who combined wisdom and compassion in a way hitherto unknown, he who realized full enlightenment by heroic self-effort, changed the course of religion, philosophy and psychology, science, art and culture in the world from which he departed two-and-a-half thousand years ago. Over the course of time he has been an inspiration and example to billions of people striving to understand themselves and the nature of existence and seeking to bring peace and goodness into their own lives and into the world. The inspiration of the Buddha remains with us, and his illumination shines with undiminished brilliance.

The Heart of Dharma

The teachings of the Buddha spread across Asia in the centuries that followed his death, and Buddhism became a world religion—the only Indian religion to achieve that status and influence. Over the course of time many different schools and traditions of Buddhism developed, and these adjusted to the cultural distinctions of their new homelands. But no matter what form of Buddhism, Zen or Pure Land,

Hinayana or Mahayana, and no matter from where, Ceylon, China or Tibet, the essence of Buddhism is the same and is summarized in the Buddha's first teaching on the Four Noble Truths.

The first truth is the truth of suffering—the inherent frustrations of conditioned existence. Everything is compounded, impermanent, bound to pass away. There are four primary sufferings: birth, sickness, old age, and death. Secondary sufferings are not getting what we want, not wanting what we get, being separated from whomever or whatever is dear to us, and being joined to people and things we dislike.

The second truth is the truth of the cause of suffering—craving, the craving for passion, the craving for existence, the craving for non-existence. Selfish craving tends to rebirth, produces samsara, and causes unhappiness to ourselves and others.

The third truth is the truth of the end of suffering—the cessation of craving, non-attachment, release, nirvana. The removal of craving allows one to go beyond—go to tranquility, to dwell in the absolute nature of stillness, unutterable blissful peace. This is not a negative state, not the cessation of awareness. Rather, it is the full awakening of awareness of reality unobscured by the deluded activity of thoughts and emotions.

The fourth truth is the truth of the path to the end of suffering—the eightfold path of right view, right intention, right speech, right action, right livelihood, right effort, right mindfulness, and right concentration. This path is summarized as the development of morality, meditation and wisdom.

There are two other basic doctrinal formulations that support this main teaching. One is the doctrine of no-self. There is no independent self-entity, no self either in ourselves or in the phenomenal world around us. There is only conditioned existence.

The sense of self which we experience is comprised of the five *skandhas,* the five aggregates or psycho-physical groupings. These are form, feeling, perception, concept, and consciousness. The first three are instinctual processes; the last two are volitional. It is the dynamic interplay of these five rather than a permanent ontological self that describes the ego-sense (and from a Buddhist point of view, one gets into trouble—strays into delusion—when this sense of self is grasped at as a solid entity rather than experienced as a changing expression of existential interaction). In terms of the world of matter and energy, the five interacting components of existence are described as the five elements: earth, fire, water, air, and space.

Since there is no inherent self-existence either of self or phenomena, the world and its creatures should be known as an illusion:

> As stars, a fault of vision, a lamp,
> A mock show, dewdrops, or a bubble,
> A dream, a lightning flash, or a cloud,
> so should we view what is conditioned.[9]

The other basic teaching is the doctrine of "conditioned co-production" (interdependent origination). As stated in the Buddhist scriptures, this formulation is as follows:

> Conditioned by Ignorance are the Karma-formations;
> conditioned by the karma-formations is Consciousness;
> conditioned by consciousness is Name and Form;
> conditioned by name and form are the Six Sense-fields;
> conditioned by the six sense-fields is Contact;
> conditioned by contact are Feelings;
> conditioned by feelings is Craving;
> conditioned by craving is Grasping;
> conditioned by grasping is Becoming;
> conditioned by becoming is Birth;
> conditioned by birth are Decay and Death, sorrow,
>   lamentation, pain, sadness and despair.
> Thus is the origination of all this mass of suffering.[10]

The reversal of the above stated links or process of conditioned co-production is the practice of Dharma leading to nirvana. The triple nature of Buddhist practice is the development of morality, concentration and wisdom, and the main support for all these practices is the cultivation of mindfulness.

The basis of Buddhist morality is the development of love, kindness, and compassion. The essence of it is to never bring harm or suffering to other beings and to try to help them and bring them happiness.

The basis of Buddhist concentration and meditation is the control of the mind. By gaining power of concentration and mindfulness we can control the wild thoughts and emotions that produce suffering and karma. The essence of this has been described as follows:

The turmoil is caused in main by three agents: (1) the senses, (2) the passions, wants and desires, and (3) discursive thinking. In order to conquer these enemies of spiritual quietude it is therefore necessary to withdraw the senses from their objects, as the tortoise draws in all its limbs; to cease from wanting anything; and to cut off discursive thinking.[11]

The development of wisdom is an intellectual and meditative understanding of the conditioned co-production and the reality of there being "no self."

The explanation of these basic Buddhist doctrines from the Tibetan or Vajrayana point of view is as follows.[12]

The source of all painful, conditioned phenomenal existence, samsara, is our acting in a state of not-seeing. It is caused by our basic ignorance or unawareness. The ground of all is actually void and luminous, beyond conception, beyond birth and death. Given a name, it is called the "Essence of Enlightenment" or the "Buddha-nature." Beings who do not recognize this primordial purity, the void luminous limitless space, fall into delusion through ignorance. Because of the karma of past tendencies, habits, and actions, the movement of mind arises in the voidness. In a fog of unawareness, holding on to the "I" even though there is no such thing, one grasps at these movements, either with greed or hatred, and thus creates the illusion of their having a separate existence. From these two—the subtle karmic forces and the inner holding onto "I"—the outer gross actions start to unfold as the five sense doors and the eight consciousnesses.

By not seeing that the movement of mind, the sense of "I" and other, is insubstantial and shares in the nature of voidness, one grasps at it as something real and thereby creates the illusion of separateness and the duality of subject and object. In this way, with the three basic mental defilements of ignorance, desire, and hatred, the mind ensnares itself. And with our constant graspings and longings we fall into a state of dissatisfaction.

From the root of these negative emotions come all physical and mental disease and suffering. The source of disease and emotionality is the lack of control of one's mind. The only way out of suffering is to uproot the basic ignorance, unawareness, that has caused our delusion and its resultant tortures. We do this through the practice of Dharma.

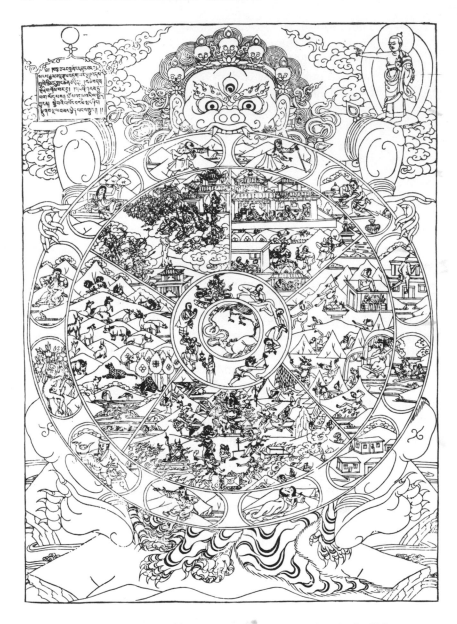

Figure 5 A pictorial representation of Buddhist teaching: the wheel of life, samsara, held in the grasp of the Lord of Death. At the hub are a pig, cock and snake, symbolizing the three mental poisons that generate the six realms of existence seen within the spokes of the wheel. Around the rim are images of the twelve links of interdependent origination, the chain of causal factors that keep samsara spinning. Tibetans say that liberation from this vicious cycle of suffering comes from the medicine of Dharma.

In order to see how the painful state of existential frustration has come about, one of the initial Dharma practices is to examine where the "I" is located. Through such analysis one discovers that the "I" cannot be found to exist anywhere, either in the body, senses or brain. One finds that the moment in which thoughts arise and are perceived as being separated from oneself is the same moment that the concept of the "I" comes about. Simultaneously, also, the grasping ensues. One begins to see that it is this dualistic subject-object grasping arising from basic unawareness that creates karma and perpetuates our delusion and suffering.

This experience helps to dissolve our tenacious grasping at ourselves and the rest of the world as solid, permanent, self-existing entities. By letting go of the ego sense, we can begin to penetrate more directly into the nature of mind and to experience stillness and voidness.

In such meditation, one simply watches the material that arises in the mind, without grasping at it or reacting to it. In this way neurotic mental patterns and emotions are recognized but at the same time their hold on the meditator is lessened. One begins to free oneself from their affect. One begins to develop true concentration and control the mind. One also begins to become aware of the stillness that exists between the arising thoughts.

All actions of body, speech, and mind that we do in a state of unawareness have an effect in accordance with the law of karma, cause and effect. This is how the universe at large and our individual situations in particular are produced. We can never meet a situation that is not the result of past karma, good or bad. The awareness or lack of awareness with which we experience the condition of the present (caused by past karma) produces the new karma that determines our future. So, far from being a fatalistic situation, our present situation is highly creative. We are free to control the state of mind and motivation we possess in the present. But we tend to act and react in unawareness; thus the force of karma tends to perpetuate the mass of unconscious habits that propel us into the cycles of existence.

The complete reversal or removal of our mental obscurations and the complete end of karma come with enlightenment. By dwelling in the absolute stillness and void that we discover between the thoughts, one comes to see that the movements of mind and the consciousness of these movements are not separate from the voidness. In this meditation one is not involved with past thoughts or chasing after future thoughts or even distracted by present thoughts. Instead, one dwells on the present, clear awareness of the voidness. Through an absolute and direct realization of the emptiness and primordial purity as Buddha-nature, one can become enlightened.

To practice Dharma, to enter the path of uprooting our ignorance, sickness, and suffering three things are said to be needed: first, to gain firmness of mind and to develop devotion; second, to be straightforward and free of deceitful thoughts; and third, to develop kindness.

To turn one's mind to the aspiration toward enlightenment, complete and ultimate health, Tibetan tradition holds that one must recognize four basic facts. Without recognizing and pondering these facts, one will never develop the intention and diligence to practice Dharma. These are (1) the preciousness of the human birth in which one can hear and practice Dharma, for such a birth is difficult to obtain; (2) the impermanence of all and everything; (3) the inevitability of the law of karma; and (4) the pervasiveness of suffering in the world of conditioned existence or samsara.

According to the Buddhists, there are six realms of beings in the world of samsara: beings in the god realm; in the demi-god or jealous god realm; in the human realm; in the animal realm; in the tortured spirits realm; and in the hell realm. Wherever one may be born in these six realms, one is always subject to impermanence, karma and suffering. Even the gods, who live long and who love the pleasure and happiness of their position, will eventually fall from that state when their karma as a god is exhausted and will take rebirth in a lower realm. Only those who achieve enlightenment will transcend the wheel of birth and death and find the complete and lasting happiness and peace that is nirvana.

There is a well known Buddhist parable that illustrates how recognition of these basic truths can be used as medicine to lead one out of self-involved suffering and onto the path.

A woman named Gotami had a young son who died. Gotami became mad with grief and sorrow, and carrying the corpse of her child on her hip, she went begging throughout the village for medicine to restore him. But no one could help her and eventually she went to the Enlightened One and asked him for medicine. The Buddha, in compassion and seeing promise in her, told her to go to a house where no one had ever died and to bring mustard-seed from it. So Gotami went from house to house, but she could not find a home or family where death had not visited. And through this her frenzy left her and she understood that no one escapes the pain of death and loss, and that Buddha had foreseen she would see this and would be comforted.

Then, bidding her dear child goodbye, she took his body to the cremation ground and cast him upon it, uttering this stanza:

> No village law, no law of market town,
> No law of single house is this—
> Of all the world and all the worlds of gods
> This only is the Law, that all things are impermanent.[13]

So saying, she returned to the Master and asked him to give her refuge. And not long afterwards, from studying the cause of things, her insight grew and she became a realized saint (arhat).

The Medical Analogy in Buddhism and the Three Yanas

The Buddha himself described his role and his teaching in terms of a fundamental medical analogy that runs throughout all forms of Buddhism. In his own lifetime, the Buddha was known as "the Great Physician" since the purpose of his teaching is to cure suffering. And over time, the Buddha became the model of the doctor-saint whom Buddhist physicians sought to emulate, the spiritually realized being who serves others by healing their ills.

The Buddhist medical analogy is clearly stated in the sutra entitled the *Lotus of the Good Law,* in which the Buddha said:

> In this comparison, the Tathagata must be regarded as a great physician; and all beings must be regarded as blinded by error, like the man born blind. Affection, hatred, error, and the sixty-two false doctrines are [the humors] wind, bile, phlegm. The four medicinal plants are these four truths: namely, the state of void, the absence of a cause, the absence of an object, and the entrance into annihilation.[14]

And in another scripture, the *Mahaparinirvana Sutra,* there are four basic motivations stated as necessary for the practice of Dharma. These are: to consider the teacher as a doctor; to consider oneself as sick; to consider the teaching as medicine; and to consider practice of the teaching as treatment.

In expounding the Four Noble Truths the Buddha described a sequence of disease and prescribed its cure. The cause of the disease, as we have discussed, is basic ignorance. This ignorance produces desire and hatred. All the specific 84,000 defilements which the Buddha described can be condensed into these "three poisons." The medicine that cures them is the three fold training that summarizes the path of Dharma. Morality cures desire, greed and lust and uses as a means of treatment the meditation on revulsion, the ugliness and disgustingness of the object of attraction. Concentration cures anger, hatred and repulsion, using the means of the meditation on compassion. Wisdom cures ignorance through the meditation on interdependent origination.

Of these, the development of wisdom (prajna) is the most important since it attacks the root poison of ignorance from which all other poisons arise. Therefore, wisdom or prajna is said to be the ultimate medicine that cures all disease and pain.

Although all schools of Buddhism rely on the Four Noble Truths and their prescription for purifying the defilements, they express the medical analogy in distinctly different ways, each appropriate to the varying philosophical views. This expanse of views reflects the enormous changes which took place in Buddhism during the more than a thousand years between the time of the Buddha and the early forms of Buddhism and the later Mahayana and tantric Buddhism that went to Tibet.

The main division in Buddhism is between the Hinayana (literally the "common vehicle") and the Mahayana (the "greater vehicle"). The Vajrayana (the "diamond vehicle") is a further advancement of the Mahayana and arose in conjunction with the development of tantra. The Buddhism of Tibet is actually a combination of all these three vehicles.

The Hinayana path, which is also called Theravadin or "the Way of the Elders," is a continuation of early Buddhism. It emphasizes renunciation, ascetic purity, and the meditation on mindfulness. Its central concept is impermanence. It relies on the teachings of the Buddha himself, organized into a three-fold collection called the Tripitaka, the "three baskets," related to the three-fold training. These include the Vinaya (morality—rules of discipline), the Sutras (meditation—the sermons of the Buddha written down after his death), and the Abhidharma (wisdom—the doctrine based on the analysis of the data of experience).

The Hinayana spiritual ideal is to achieve liberation for oneself. It is embodied in the figure of the arhat who reaches the quiesence of nirvana and becomes exempt from the rounds of birth and death. This, however, does not imply a state of complete Buddhahood, but rather of sainthood.

In the Hinayana, the medical prescription in terms of the three poisons is simple: keep them away. The Hinayana practice is to tame the mind by controlling the passion-poisons and to withdraw from the world where those poisons predominate. In general, the Hinayana path emphasizes practicing the medicine of renunciation to cure the sickness of desire (rather than hatred or ignorance).

The Mahayana spiritual ideal is to achieve liberation for the sake of other beings. It is embodied in the concept of the bodhisattva. The bodhisattva, out of love for all beings, tiny bugs and kings equally, vows to put off his own entrance into nirvana so that he may stay in the world to liberate all other beings from suffering before himself. The bodhisattva vow and ideal is the path of love. This is expressed most beautifully by the Indian Buddhist poet-saint Shantideva:

> As long as the existence of space and
> as long as the existence of the world,
> that long let my existence be
> devoted to the world's sorrows.
>
> Whatever the sorrow of the world,
> may all that ripen in me;
> and may the world be
> comforted by the glorious Bodhisattvas.[15]

The bodhisattva path is to develop wisdom by recognizing the emptiness of self and others and to generate active love and compassion as the expression of that wisdom. The Mahayana is grounded in awakening the "thought of enlightenment," the bodhicitta, the aspiration to perfection for the sake of all beings, since Buddhahood, full enlightenment, is said to exist inherently in all sentient beings but to be obscured by their defilements.

The Mahayana teaches that the intrinsic Buddha-nature is realized gradually over successive lifetimes by practicing the career of a bodhisattva—developing wisdom and compassion together. By realizing the true nature of phenomena (wisdom) and by generating

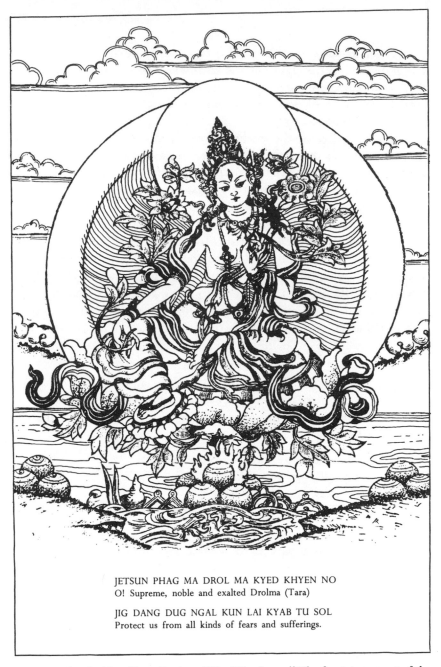

JETSUN PHAG MA DROL MA KYED KHYEN NO
O! Supreme, noble and exalted Drolma (Tara)

JIG DANG DUG NGAL KUN LAI KYAB TU SOL
Protect us from all kinds of fears and sufferings.

Figure 6 The Goddess Tara, Drolma, "She Who Saves." The feminine aspect of the Buddha-nature, Tara symbolizes the wisdom of emptiness and is thus renowned as the "Mother of All the Buddhas." She is invoked for protection from all kinds of sickness; all the goddesses of medicine are her emanations. The short prayer shown here was received from Tara in a vision by the 19th century lama, Dudjom Lingpa.

the thought of enlightenment for oneself and others (compassion), the bodhisattva eventually becomes a Buddha.

The bodhicitta, the thought of enlightenment, is said to be the one great thought that always bears positive fruit. As inspiration and motivation, it is awakened by the practice of the "four boundless meditations": boundless love, boundless compassion, boundless sympathetic joy and boundless equanimity. The open, endless nature of these positive qualities, generated from the heart, leads to a state of complete meditative absorption *(samadhi)*.

As activity, the bodhicitta is developed through the practice of the "six perfections": generosity, morality, patience, strenuousness, meditation and wisdom. The first, generosity, is the beginning of the path of non-attached action. It is said that we may begin to develop it simply by practicing giving from one of our own hands to the other. Each successive perfection *(paramita)* is vaster than the previous one and incorporates it. And all lead successively to wisdom—the realization that the nature of phenomena is emptiness.

Emptiness, *shunyata,* is the central concept of the Mahayana. Shunyata expresses the nature of absolute reality, and the realization of shunyata or emptiness is the wisdom aspect of the Mahayana. The deep meaning of the void is summarized in the Buddhist literature called the *Perfection of Wisdom* or the *Prajna-Paramita Sutra,* but the concept of emptiness, because of its very nature, is hard to describe. As it says in the *Prajna-Paramita Sutra,* "Shunyata is the synonym of that which has no cause, that which is beyond thought or conception, that which is not produced, that which is not born, that which is without measure."[16]

There is really no adequate word in English for shunyata, as both "voidness" and "emptiness" have negative connotations, whereas shunyata is a positive sort of emptiness transcending the duality of positive-negative. The doctrine of the void was propounded in the Madhyamika dialectic philosophy of Nagarjuna, the second-century Indian Buddhist philosopher-saint. Nagarjuna said of shunyata, "It cannot be called void or not void, or both or neither, but in order to indicate it, it is called the Void."[17]

This shunyata can be understood intellectually from philosophy and life experience, but to realize it deeply as the true reality of non-duality, in the sense that our awareness expands into the space of its radiant openness, we must experience it in deep meditation. Through such meditative realization of emptiness, one can become enlightened.

The absolute compassion of the Mahayana arises spontaneously with the realization of emptiness. Since we all share the nature of emptiness, how can we bear the suffering of others, all the beings who have at one time or another been our mothers (and brothers, enemies, lovers, etc.) in the endless cycles of rebirth caused by egotistic ignorance and grasping at the illusion of duality.

In the medical analogy of the general Mahayana, love and compassion is the medicine that cures the sickness of hatred and anger. In the higher Mahayana, shunyata is the ultimate medicine. Emptiness is the antidote for all poisons and defilements. Therefore, there is no need to withdraw from the world to be cured of its poisons. In fact, the love and compassion of the Mahayana demands that the bodhisattva stay in the world of passions in order to help other beings.

Since Buddhahood is immanent in all beings and can be realized though awareness of shunyata, it follows that the whole phenomenal universe can be perceived in terms of its intrinsic Buddha-nature and thus be seen to be populated with innumerable Buddhas and bodhisattvas who exist in cosmic "pure lands" beyond the realm of dualistic experience.

According to the Mahayana there are infinite Buddhas, bodhisattvas and deities. They represent various aspects of the absolute Buddha-nature. For example, Avalokitesvara is the compassion aspect, Manjushri is the wisdom aspect, and Vajrapani is the power aspect. The goddess Tara embodies the inspiration of emptiness and is the female aspect of Buddha-nature. Vaidurya Guru or the Medicine Buddha embodies the healing aspect.

It is in the Mahayana that the Medicine Buddha first appears, and veneration of the Lord of Healing became one of the most popular and widespread devotional "cults" in Mahayana. The Medicine Buddha was worshipped as the dispenser of spiritual medicine that could cure spiritual, psychological and physical disease. Among the twelve vows that the Medicine Buddha is believed to have taken is that of curing just by the hearing of his name or the thought of him. His sheer existence emphasizes the importance of healing in the Mahayana.

Although the Mahayana is distinctly different in emphasis and character from the Hinayana, it still stands on the foundation of the Hinayana; it incorporates it and elaborates on it. Similarly, the Vajrayana includes and elaborates on the Mahayana.

To the Hinayana path of renunciation the Mahayana adds the path of bodhicitta, compassion; and to the Hinayana view of interdependent causation, the Mahayana adds the Madhyamika theory of voidness. The Vajrayana includes all of these but emphasizes the awakening of wisdom through the transformative energy of the phenomena that have arisen from voidness and are in fact inseparable from it.

The Vajrayana description of enlightenment reflects this different view. It is not the rejection of samsara and the goal of nirvana as in the Hinayana, nor the separate co-existence of samsara and nirvana as found in the Mahayana, but the enlightenment that is the union of samsara and nirvana in pure present awareness.

In the Vajrayana, emptiness is no longer applied as an antidote. All phenomena, self and others (relative truth) share the nature of this emptiness (absolute truth). The two truths are inseparable. To realize the luminous void ground nature is to dissolve the distinction between samsara and nirvana. Thus, all phenomena are perceived with "pure perception" as being inseparable from radiant emptiness and hence as the sacred expression of Buddha-nature. In this way, oneself and all the beings become the deities of the mandala.

The meditative recognition of emptiness is direct and blissful, and all manifestation is perceived as the play of the deity, of emptiness. There is great joy in this, great relaxation. As the Vajrayana master Longchen Rabjampa said:

> Since Mind-as-such—pure from the beginning and with no root to hold to something other than itself—has nothing to do with an agent or something to be done, one's mind may well be happy. . . . Since everything is but an apparition perfect in being what it is, having nothing to do with good or bad, acceptance or rejection, one may well burst out in laughter.[18]

In the Vajrayana the ideal is to attain Buddhahood in this very lifetime, as opposed to the gradual path of the Mahayana. The transformation from delusion to enlightenment, Buddhahood, is achieved through the practice of tantra and through the direct recognition of the Buddha-nature.

In tantra practice, the dualistic forces and manifestations are united in a way of being that transcends duality or conceptualization. Our limited and egotistical view is transformed into pure perception of phenomena as the radiant manifestation of emptiness. The means are both the yogic practices involved in the transformation of subtle energies within the body and mind and the meditation that goes directly to the penetration of absolute truth, of "Mind as such," the naked perception of the "true nature."

To explain the deep meaning of the Vajrayana, the principal metaphor used is that of the vajra. Vajra is a Sanskrit word (in Tibetan it is "dorje," *rdor-je*) meaning diamond, thunderbolt or sceptre. The inherent Buddha-nature is said to be like a diamond, indestructible, pure and empty in itself, but luminous in reflecting the manifestation of energies as rainbow light.

In tantric ritual symbolism, the vajra is the ritual sceptre that represents the essence of awakened awareness and the compassion and skillful means arising from it. The vajra's counterpart is the ritual bell that symbolizes emptiness and the wisdom and bliss inherent in it. The union of these two represents absolute enlightenment, the self-liberated Buddha-nature of all phenomena.

According to the Vajrayana, all esoteric enlightenment teaching originates from the Primordial Buddha. He is named Samantabhadra (Tib: Kuntuzangpo, the "'All Good'') or Vajradhara (Tib: Dorjechang, the "Diamond Holder''). This primordial inherent level of truth is called Dharmakaya, Thatness, Buddha-essence.

Our true nature is identical with the Primordial Buddha, but due to our obscurations we have forgotten our true nature and so wander in samsara. The example is often given that our true nature is like the sky—open, spacious, unending and unbeginning. Our mental defilements and obscurations are like clouds. The purpose of the tantric Buddhist practices is to remove and transform the obscurations so that we rediscover and realize our Buddha-identity.

In order to communicate the absolute truth to those who cannot perceive it for themselves, the Primordial Buddha, out of compassion, manifests an uncountable number of manifestations in all realms and on all levels. Because of the needs of different kinds of beings, the one hundred wrathful and peaceful deities are manifested.

From the primordial abiding truth represented by the Adi-Buddha springs forth a five-fold division of Dhyani Buddhas representing the Buddha-nature of the manifested cosmos. These are the active and subtle manifestations sprung from the unmanifest radiant space of emptiness. This is the Sambhogakaya level. The Dhyani Buddhas are pictured in a mandala, a circular cosmogram demonstrating the radiation of Buddha-nature. Each one represents a specific dynamic wisdom, enlightenment quality, faculty, direction, sound, color, gesture, etc. Tantric and Mahayana Buddhism have many arrangements of Buddhas, deities, and bodhisattvas emanating from the basic mandala of the five Dhyani Buddhas.

When the Buddha-nature manifests on the gross, material plane, such as the historical Buddha Shakyamuni, it is called the Nirmanakaya level.

Thus the three kayas, the "three bodies of the Buddha," the Dharmakaya, the Sambhogakaya and the Nirmanakaya represent the Buddhist sacred trinity of the three levels of expression of the reality of Buddha-nature. They represent the unmanifest, subtle and manifest levels of Buddha-essence. They represent the Buddha mind, the Buddha speech, and the Buddha body.

In Vajrayana, the practice is to transform ourselves and the world around us into the body, speech and mind of the Buddha. These practices are described in a series of texts known as tantras (Tibetan *rgyud*). Through tantric esoteric rituals the practitioner creates and simultaneously identifies with a particular form of deity. This is accomplished through visualization, mantras (special formulas of syllables that use the spiritual power of sound vibration), mudras (symbolic gestures that awaken spiritual receptivity and awareness), and through formless meditation.

In these tantric sadhanas or, in fact, in any meditation or religious practice, there are three things the tradition holds of main importance; first, to have the intention of doing the practice for the sake of the liberation of all beings; second, to be unattached to the experiences that may arise in meditation; and third, to share the merit of the practice, to dedicate the seeds of awareness and the good karma created in the practice to the universal womb of illumination.

In the Vajrayana, the guru or lama takes on a special and central significance because he can, through the power of his enlightened awareness, introduce the disciple to the nature of his own mind or true reality. This is called a direct mind-to-mind transmission. The guru performs special empowerments or initiations in which he introduces the disciple to the mandala of the deity and brings him or her face to face with the illumination of reality.

The disciple may or may not be able to maintain this awareness after the initiation, but the seed of illumination has been planted. If the disciple practices the sadhana according to the instruction and with the right intention and diligence, it can result in enlightenment. Therefore, in the Vajrayana the guru is of supreme importance.

A Tibetan lama has explained it this way:

> All the Buddhas have the desire to aid us. But we are not able to see them or communicate with them—as we do with the Guru.
>
> Dorje Chang, Vajradhara, and Samantabhadra are all names of Buddha, of all Buddhas. Vajra (diamond) is indestructible; since all the Buddhas have unveiled their minds of klesha (mental defilements), the spirit of all the Buddhas is indestructible, like the vajra. The Guru is the essence of Vajradhara. . . . [19]

In all the Buddhist yanas, the basic practice is refuge, to take refuge in the Triple Gem of the Buddha, the Dharma and the Sangha. This is like admitting one is ill and taking the support of the doctor and his medicine. In the Vajrayana, two more triple refuges are added to this basic one.

The first is refuge in the guru, the meditation deity (the yidam— the specific form and aspect of Buddha-nature), and the feminine wisdom (the dakini, Tibetan "khandroma," "the sky going mother"), the sensuous aspect of voidness.

The second additional refuge is in the *tri-kaya,* the "Three bodies of Buddha." The Dharmakaya (Tib: *chos-sku*) is called the absolute truth body, Buddha-mind, unborn, undying all-pervasive voidness. The Sambhogakaya (*longs-sku*) is called enjoyment body, Buddha speech, the energetic rainbow-like subtle level. The Nirmanakaya (*sprul-sku*) is called the form body, Buddha body, and is characterized by the unobstructed action of compassion.

To recognize and realize these "three bodies" in oneself is the goal of Vajrayana practice, the result of transforming one's own physical, psycho-mental and spiritual energies through tantric practices. This is also the goal of tantric medicine, as will be described in the section on tantric healing.

As far as the medical analogy is concerned, in the Vajrayana the poisons are neither kept away nor cured with the antidote of emptiness. Instead the poisons are used as medicines, transformed into "nectar" by recognition of their Buddha-nature. The example is often given of the peacock who eats poison and thrives on it in splendor. The meaning of this is that the energies of habitual thought and conflicted emotion are identified with the wisdom ground of voidness from which they arise. Thus, the poisons are liberated upon arising by unwavering, diamond-like awareness and in this way their energy becomes "medicine," food for awareness and hence realization.

In the higher Mahayana and Vajrayana, the Medicine Buddha is not simply worshipped for his healing powers. The Medicine Buddha is the form of Buddha-nature that the practitioner aspires to realize in himself. Through practice of meditation on the Medicine Buddha, one can generate enormous healing power for self-healing and for the healing of others. Thus, the exalted model that the Tibetan Buddhist physician aspires to emulate is none other than the Medicine Buddha himself. While the physician is practicing medicine normally, he is spiritually identified with the Medicine Buddha.

Vajrayana Buddhism was developed in India by the great tantric sages, the *maha-siddhas,* and is the diamond Buddhism that was established in Tibet. A tantric orientation effected everything Tibetan, and this is no less true of Tibetan medicine than Tibetan Buddhism. Without attempting to give a complete outline of the Tantrayana, the few salient features presented above help orient us in the study of Tibetan Buddhist medicine and psychiatry, for tantric Buddhism is the well-spring of Tibet's healing waters.

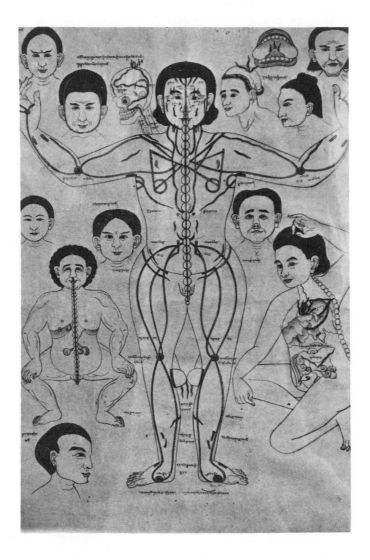

Figure 7 Tibetan medical chart showing the blood vessels and points for blood-letting, the placement of internal organs, and a variety of head and facial shapes corresponding to humoral body and character types.

3

Indian Medicine and Buddhism

Ayurveda

Tibetan medicine is based on the traditional medical system of India, Ayurveda, literally "the science of long life." Ayurveda is a holistic system aimed at managing life in such a way as to prolong it and prevent disease.

Ayurveda is a sacred science. According to Indian mythology, it was first perceived by the god Brahma. From Brahma it was passed on to the fabulous mythical Ashwin twins, to the god Indra, and finally to Atreya, a human. Atreya taught medicine at the ancient metropolis of Taxila. His six main students, in turn, scattered over India and spread the teaching.

The beginning of Ayurveda as an actual medical tradition dates from the Vedic period in the middle of the second millenium B.C. The *Rig Veda,* the earliest known Indian literature, mentions various maladies and notes the attempts of people to cure them. This ancient scripture also contains a complete hymn to magical and medicinal plants.

It is the *Atharva Veda,* however, which is the earliest source of therapeutic prescriptions that began the Ayurvedic tradition. Basically, the *Atharva Veda* equates disease with the influence of demons. It prescribes magical and herbal medicine—a variety of plants, charms and incantations—to ward off the evil spells of demons and enemies and to improve health and sexual vigor.

While magic and religion were inextricably mixed with medicine in the Vedic period, an independent medical tradition was developing and with it the emergence of a class of professional physicians as distinct from the earlier priest-magician healers. But it is also true that in the Vedic period it was the prophet-poets or rishis who, from their meditation and heightened powers of yogic observation, learned to heal and preserve their own and other's bodies and thus enlarged and developed the medical tradition.

The second and classical stage of Ayurveda's development began with the Brahmanical period in 800 B.C., reached its finest heights in the early centuries A.D., and continued as an unbroken tradition until the Moslem conquest of India in the 13th century.

During this second stage, Ayurveda became a rational or scientific medical system wonderfully advanced for its time. Some of its medical discoveries and techniques, plastic surgery for example, were not known in the West until thousands of years later.

At the beginning of this classical period, the medical teaching was still entirely oral, but by the first century A.D. the written tradition had grown remarkably, a reflection of the enormous medical knowlege that was being codified, refined and further developed. By the third century there was written evidence of a "thriving Indian therapy." A fragment of *Indica,* a report of a third century Greek who traveled the Ganges River, is part of this record:

> [The physicians] know how to make women fertile and how these can give birth to boys or girls, by employing drugs. They heal diseases usually by ordering suitable foods and not by use of medicines. Mostly they employ drugs as cataplasms or by rubbing into the skin because other means are not free of undesirable effects.[20]

Classical Ayurveda was divided into eight branches of medicine:
1. surgery *(salya)*
2. treatment of disorders of the head and neck *(salakya)*
3. general medicine or therapy of the organism *(kayacikitsa)*
4. psychiatry or mental diseases caused by demons *(bhuta-vidya)*
5. pediatrics—childhood diseases caused by demons *(kaumara-bhutya)*
6. toxicology—medical drugs for poisons *(agada)*
7. rejuvenation, elixirs *(rasayana)*
8. virilification *(vajikarana,* lit. "turning into a stallion")

Within these eight branches the Vedic approach persists, that is the religious element and the psychosomatic view. But to that approach was added a rational or scientific approach, "the rational use of naturalistic theories to organize and interpret systematic empirical observations."[21] The rational view of the body in disease and health was expressed in terms of a humoral theory of medicine. Exactly what—if any—relationship there is between the development of Indian Ayurvedic humoral medicine and the classical Greek system of humoral medicine has not yet been established by scholars.

The three humors (*doshas,* literally "faults") are air, bile and phlegm. They are simply understood as the underlying constituents of the body, but as Heinrich Zimmer has explained, they are in fact "not just airy, bilious and mucous matter found in the body but three principles of life-energy."[22]

All Ayurvedic therapy was accompanied by prayer. Treatment aimed at restoring humoral balance was prescribed through food and herbs classified according to "six tastes," "five elements," "ten qualities" etc. Preventive medicine and hygiene were emphasized and these included toothbrushing, massage and even politeness. Diagnosis was based on questioning and inspection, but prognosis was a more mystical matter of divination by dreams and omens.

At its high point of development, Ayurvedic doctors practiced excellent surgery, the most advanced of its time, and were famous for plastic surgery and removal of cataracts. It has been said by medical historians that they had good clinical knowlege, recognized blood-spitting in pulmonary tuberculosis, knew leprosy was contagious and made excellent descriptions of epileptic and convulsive disorders. They were also, it has been noted, obsessed with classifications (sixty diseases of the oral cavity), preferentially concerned with the preservation of the male species, and tended, as time went on, to include everything in their herbal medicines that had ever been suggested.

The three most famous figures in classical Ayurveda were Sushruta, Charaka, and Vagbhata. Sushruta and Charaka both wrote encyclopedic medical treatises called *samhitas.* The *Charaka Samhita* was based on an earlier and now lost samhita by Agnivesa, a student of Atreya. Charaka's work has survived to our time. It contains the comprehensive theory and knowledge of Ayurveda, summarizing the ancient oral medical tradition in the form of lessons. Zimmer has stated that it "stands as the finest [medical] document of the creative period of the last centuries before the beginning of our era, both in regard to the extent of its contents and to its state of preservation."[23]

The other great early figure of Ayurveda was Sushruta. He compiled the *Sushruta Samhita,* a comprehensive work that especially details the practice of Indian surgery, which was, as already noted, highly advanced. Both Charaka and Sushruta probably lived in the final centuries B.C. Scholarly controversy abounds on the subject of their dates, but it is quite certain that both of them lived somewhere between the sixth century B.C. and the second century A.D.[24] The third great figure in classical Ayurveda was Vagbhata, and he can be said with some certainty to have lived in the seventh century A.D.

Buddhism's Influence on Ayurveda

Vagbhata was a Buddhist, and his work clearly shows the influence of Buddhist ethics on Indian medicine. In the introductory stanza of his medicine manual he pays homage "to that unique physician" the Buddha "who rooted out and removed all diseases like lust, and so on, which cause delusion and indolence, and are spread over all living beings, sticking to them always."[25] Vaghbata devotes an entire chapter of his book to the relation of health to morals, advocating the development of a mental attitude of unselfish affection as a potential health-giver. He exhorted physcians to practice the Buddha's compassion and treat all beings, even worms and ants, as equal to oneself.

A number of Western scholars have noted the positive influence of Buddhism on Ayurveda, and, in fact, the high period or golden age of Ayurveda corresponds with the period of Buddhism's ephemeral glory in India (from approximately the middle of the fourth century B.C. to the middle of eighth century A.D.), also the period when India's and Buddhism's influence spread abroad.

While Ayurveda is sometimes called Hindu medicine, it became, during that period, just as equally Buddhist medicine. As one scholar noted, "Buddhism, which encouraged the virtue of compassion and was less bound than Hinduism by considerations of ritual purity, seems to have been particularly conducive to the study of medicine. . . . The Buddha himself was interested in medicine and laid down many rules and regulations for the care and treatment of sick monks."[26]

The Buddha knew Ayurveda well. As Zimmer has pointed out, "The Buddha, in expounding his doctrine of salvation, modeled it after the attitude of the Hindu physician toward the task of healing."[27]

An Ayurvedic doctor was taught to regard a patient and the sickness in this sequence: 1. Is there a disease and if so, what is it? 2.

What is the cause of the disease? 3. Is there a cure for the disease? 4. If the disease is curable, what is the proper treatment? We recognize this sequence as that used by the Buddha in expounding the essence of Dharma, the Four Noble Truths.

That the Buddha's first and central teaching should be linked to India's great medical tradition in such a basic way serves to emphasize that the medical analogy in Buddhism is not simply a metaphor in words but is a vital aspect of Buddhism. If at the beginning Buddhism and medicine were so intimately connected, then it is not surprising that Ayurveda flourished in India with the rise of Buddhism there and was later brought to Tibet with the establishment of Dharma.

The Buddha instructed his monks on necessary medical procedures for them to take if the standard "seven-limbs of enlightenment" (mindfulness, striving, tranquilty, etc.) had not produced a cure. In the medicine section of the Vinaya he noted that certain foods, such as honey and butter, should be taken as medicines by the monks; in fact, he prescribed many different vegetable, animal, and mineral substances as remedies for ill monks. However, the Blessed One prohibited the practice of medicine outside the monastic order, specifically prohibiting the monks from earning a livelihood as healers.

Among his lay followers, however, there were doctors, and among these was the Buddha's personal physician, Jivaka. Jivaka's greatness as a doctor and surgeon became legendary in India. His supreme skill as a physician was matched by his supreme devotion to Lord Buddha, whom he attended three times a day. The Buddha declared Jivaka to be chief among his lay followers. Because of his medical eminence, Jivaka was three times crowned in public as "King of Doctors," and he is therefore known as the "Thrice Crowned Physician."

The influence of the Buddha's "moral genius" on Ayurveda during his own time and in succeeding centuries has been described by the Indian writer Mitra:

> Compassion was the source of his morality and the good of all the goal of his moral conduct. Under the moral conducts, the inclusion of celibacy, knowledge, charity, amicableness, compassion, joy, impartiality, and peace in Ayurveda is positively influenced by Buddhism.[28]

With the spread of Buddhism went the spread of Ayurveda and the influence Buddhism had on it. Two hundred years after the

Buddha, the Emperor of India, Ashoka, converted to Buddhism and began a remarkable reign of peace and humanitarian government. Among his many social ordinances, evidence of which remain to this day in the form of stone pillars on which the message of the ordinance was chiseled, was one on medicine. It concerned the establishment of hospitals for both humans and animals and the cultivation of medicine plants. The II Rock Edict of Ashoka states:

> These [medical centers] consist of the medical care of man and the care of animals. Medicinal herbs whether of use to man or to beast have been brought and planted wherever they did not grow; similarly, roots and fruits have been brought and planted wherever they did not grow. Along the roads wells have been dug and trees planted for the use of men and beasts.[29]

Ashoka's hospitals predated similar institutions in the West by many centuries. During Ashoka's reign the practice of Ayurveda thrived and reached to the far corners of his enormous empire—from

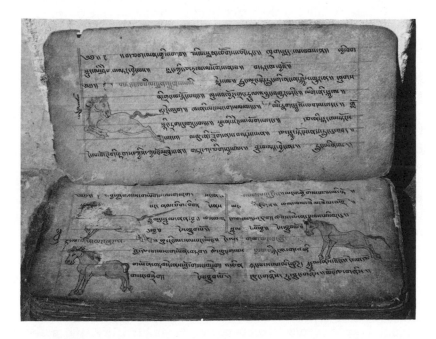

Figure 8 Ancient, handwritten, illustrated Tibetan veterinary text. The care of animals was emphasized by Buddhism, and Indian Ayurveda developed veterinary science. The major Ayurvedic work on horse medicine was translated into Tibetan by Rinchen Zangpo.

Afghanistan to Ceylon to the Western frontiers of the Greek kings, where Ashoka also built thousands of monasteries and Buddhist shrines.

Another example of a benevolent Buddhist king who took a great interest in medicine and the health of his subjects was the fourth century Ceylonese king Buddhadasa. The king, who had studied medicine and even wrote a medical treatise, carried medical instruments with him wherever he went and treated his subjects, including untouchables and animals. He appointed and supported resident doctors in the villages and opened asylums for the crippled and blind.

In the Mahayana, medicine became one of the five major subjects a monk was required to study and master. Therefore, the Mahayana Buddhist tradition produced many great doctors who made significant advancements in Ayurveda.

It was in the Mahayana that the devotional worship of the Medicine Buddha, *Bhaishajyaguru,* "the Master of Healing," became prevalent. As Mahayana Buddhism spread throughout the Far East, it took Ayurveda, as one of its main sciences, and the worship of the Medicine Buddha with it. The spread of the Mahayana to China, Japan, and the Indianized kingdoms of Southeast Asia had a benevolent effect on public health. In the Khmer kingdom, now Kampuchea, hospitals were established as late as 1186 under the spiritual guardianship of the Medicine Buddha.

In China, which of course had its own marvelous medical system (whose theory of the five elements is taken from Buddhism), the spread of the Mahayana continued the Buddhist influence "in a system of medical assistance which included hospitals, leper wards and dispensaries in the larger monasteries, and which were supported by income from 'compassion fields.' This system was secularized towards the middle of the ninth century. In this way Chinese medicine acquired ethical principles of the highest order."[30]

In India itself, Ayurveda took on the distinct tone of the "Great Vehicle" as the Mahayana developed. Ayurvedic works from that period reflect this Buddhist influence. In Vagbhata's works he mentions Buddhist dieties that may be invoked for healing and proclaims that leprosy may be cured through the worship of the goddess Tara, "She who Saves." Even in contemporary India there is an Ayurvedic medicine that bears Tara's name (*Tara Mandura*).

A first century A.D. Ayurvedic text called *Sukhavativyuha,* to take another example, refers to Avalokitesvara, the bodhisattva of compassion, in his special healing manifestation as Simhananda, the "Lion-Voiced One," and credits him with being the destroyer of all diseases. Again, an Ayurvedic remedy of modern India carries his name.

Perhaps nothing better illustrates the union of religion and medicine in Buddhism and the influence of the union on Ayurveda than the fact that the greatest of the Mahayana philospher-saints were also great physicans who wrote important medical works. They made major contributions to Ayurvedic literature during its golden age.

Foremost among these is none other than Nagarjuna, the founder of the Madhyamika critical dialectic, the doctrine and philosophy of the void, upon which the entire higher Mahayana and Vajrayana teachings are based.

Nagarjuna was born a Brahmin in the "Coconut Country" (South India) in the first century A.D. The Buddhists believe that he was an incarnation of Manjushri, the wisdom aspect of the Buddha, and indeed, as a child, it is recorded that he mastered all the Vedas including magic and medicine. After his conversion to Buddhism, he continued his mastery of medicine and wrote *The Hundred Prescriptions,* as well as many other medicine works including *The Precious Collection.*

We can only wonder, in a kind of awe, at the profound greatness and scope of a being like Nagarjuna, tantric adept, philosopher, poet, master of traditional and alchemical medicine. The meditational and philosophic clarity, toned by compassion, which he brought to the study of medicine reminds us once again that the type we may call "physician-sage" is both the ideal and the source of "holistic" medicine. Such a tradition continued Nagarjuna's line.

One disciple, also a renowned Hindu pandit who converted to Buddhism, was Ashvaghosha.[31] Again, Ashvaghosha's eminence as a Buddhist philospher and poet was matched by his medical authority. He wrote three very important Ayurvedic works: *The Great Eight Branches; Entering The Eight Branches;* and *Collection of the Essence of the Eight Branches,* plus a commentary on the latter. Ashvaghosha's disciple Chandranandana wrote a commentary on his teacher's works, a dictionary of its medical terms, and major volumes of his own.

It was this same Chandranandana who wrote down in Sanskrit the teaching of the *Gyu-zhi* or *Four-Tantras* and gave it to the Tibetan translator Vairochana on the occasion of the latter's pilgrimage to India. Here we can see that the original *Gyu-zhi,* which was to become the heart-essence text of Tibetan medicine, is a continuation of the classical Ayurveda advanced by the Indian Buddhist siddhas.

The Hinayana traditions of meditation and yoga developed onwards from the time of the Buddha also produced concomitant medical insight. A work from the 4th century, the *Visuddhimagga* of Buddha-ghosa, illustrates the effect of yogic knowledge on medicine. According to Mitra: "An advanced anatomy is referred to . . . and the description of ten kinds of dead bodies, thirty-two aspects of the body including viscera. Osteology is very vividly described in the above work of Buddhist Yoga not known, so far, to the scholars of the history of Medicine."[32]

This knowledge of anatomy probably arose from the practice of examining dead bodies as a support for pondering impermanence and interdependent origination (if you look at a bone and check backwards step by step how it arrived at that condition, you may discover the twelve interdependent links). Also, Buddhist monks often recited the names of the thirty-two "disgusting" parts of the body as an antidote to lust and attachment.

As a further development of the high Mahayana, Buddhist tantra is called Vajrayana, the "diamond vehicle." The psycho-physical spiritual exercises of tantric yoga, which survive today in the Tibetan tradition, emerge from its view of the human body as a microcosm of the universe. Thus the body itself becomes venerable, transformed by tantric practice into the pure land of the Buddha. The highly developed external cosmology of Mahayana Buddhism became, in tantric practice, a diagram of sacred reality seen inside oneself.

The psycho-physical practices of tantric yoga aim at unifying the polarized universal forces as experienced within the body-mind organism. On the basis of this identification of the body with the energies of the cosmos arose a whole separate category of healing called tantric medicine.

The ancient alchemical traditions of India prospered simultaneously with tantra. Indian alchemy is obviously related to tantra as well as to medicine in that its aim is transformation of energy. The goal is to transmute the body and make it "immortal" by the use of various medicinal and "magical" herbs and substances. These are applied in conjunction with religious techniques like mantras and incantations. In this way the elements in the body become purified and transformed into their subtle counterparts.

The most important substance that alchemy relies on is mercury. Before it can be used, the highly toxic mercury must be purified and "fixed." To transform mercury in this way was one of the main problems of alchemy. For it was said of mercury that it was like the mind: by nature unsteady; but when stabilized, then there was nothing in the world that could not be accomplished. Medicine works, the *Rasaratnakara,* for example, describe it as the most powerful agent for subduing every sickness and improving bodily vigor. The preparation of mercury formed the core of this "siddha medicine," the medical techniques of the realized adepts (a siddha is a tantric adept, while *siddhi* is psychic, spiritual or "miraculous" power.)

The alchemical formulas of tantric medicine are used in the regular Tibetan medical system as elixirs and essence-pills—especially those which are mercury based—relied on for strengthening the ailing organism and for a variety of medical purposes. Additionally, yogis use these essence-nutriment pills to sustain their lives for long periods, thereby overcoming the need to eat.

Tantra elevated the role of the body in a way hitherto unknown. Tantric yoga is the esoteric inner union of religion and medicine, the internalization of ritual symbolism through which the body can be realized on its supreme level. Saraha, the tantric Buddhist siddha and poet, is well known for his radical position against the excessive outer ritualism which had developed in the Buddhism of his time. In the following verses, he expresses the splendid inner visions of the tantric adept.

> When the mind goes to rest, the bonds of the body are destroyed,
> And when the one flavour of the Innate pours forth,
> There is neither outcaste nor Brahmin.
>
> Here is the sacred Yamuna and here the River Ganges,
> Here are Prayaga and Banares, here are Sun and Moon,
> Here I have visited in my wanderings shrines and such places of pilgrimage,
> For I have not seen another shrine blissful like my own body.[33]

Thus advancements and contributions were made to Ayurvedic medicine during the civilization of Buddhist India, from the time of the Buddha in the sixth century B.C. through the development of high Mahayana and tantra a thousand years later. So it was Indian Ayurveda at its high point of development and knowledge that was methodically taken to Tibet, where the works were translated, preserved, and kept alive to generate new offspring with indigenous Tibetan contributions to medical science.

Even as late as the eleventh century, the saintly ascetic and scholar Atisha, on making his way to Tibet from his native Bengal at an advanced age, took with him his important medical work *The Heart of Life*. Thus as Mahayana and tantric Buddhism were transplanted to Tibet, so was Indian Ayurveda. Buddhism in India continued to contribute to the native medical science until the very end when, by the thirteenth century, Buddhism had completely disapperaed from India, not only the living religion but also the shrines, temples, and universities, the arts, science, and culture that represented it. The invading Moslems systematically destroyed every vestige of Buddhism which they could find, that is true. But Buddhism as a religion had already been on the decline in India for five hundred years after a thousand years of ascendancy. Much of the essence survived there, however, through its influence on Indian thought—Yoga and Vedanta, for example. As for Indian Ayurveda, it underwent a change and decline at the hands of the Moslems. Its tradition was interrupted and partly lost.

But on the snowy plateaus of Tibet, a country that came to be known as the "Land of the Healing Art," the ancient medical wisdom survived.

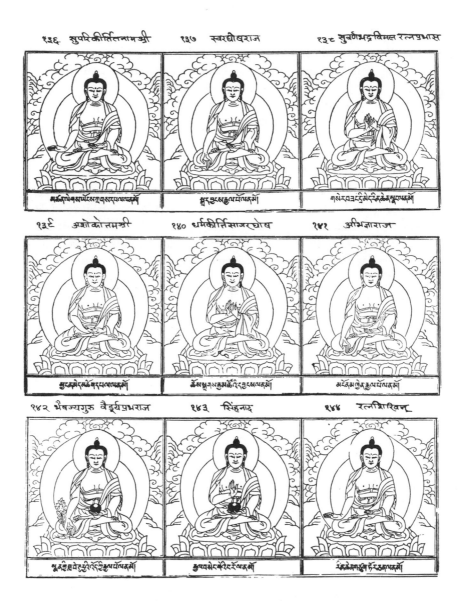

Figure 9 The Medicine Buddhas are sometimes numbered nine, as seen here in this representation from the "Three Hundred Icons of Tibet." Shakyamuni is in the middle of the bottom row in his healing form as the Lion-Voiced Buddha. To his right is the main Medicine Buddha, the King of Lapis Lazuli Light.

4

Medicine in Tibet

The Sacred Origins and the Medicine Buddha

According to the Tibetans, all medical knowledge has a sacred origin and is ascribed to the wisdom of the Buddhas. The Tibetan story of the origin of medicine is similar to the Indian one, but instead of originating from Brahma, as it does in the Hindu system, it originates from a past Buddha of a previous time cycle who had taught it to Brahma in the first place.

The Buddha who taught medicine to Brahma was the Buddha Kashyapa, the third in a line of Buddhas for our universe and the one who preceded Shakyamuni Buddha. But that was long ago in a far distant time cycle. According to Buddhist mythology, in an early part of our present time cycle (which has four division or *yugas*) human beings lived absorbed in states of deep meditation, had miraculous powers, emitted light from their bodies, and didn't even need to eat. But one day, due to the force of previous karma, a bit of bitumen fell to the ground and one man picked it up and ate it. He became sick.

Thus, indigestion was the first disease and heralded the end of the golden age. The god Brahma, learning of the man's sickness, felt compassion and wanted to cure him. Instantaneously, Brahma remembered a medicine teaching of Kashyapa Buddha—that boiling water cures digestive ailments.[34] He prescribed it. The man was cured. And medicine in our time cycle had begun.

Later, though a confluence of events, Brahma remembered the whole science of medicine that Kashyapa Buddha had taught him. He passed this medical knowledge on to the Ashwin twins, and eventually it came down to the human world and to Atreya, the famous teacher of Ayurveda at Taxila. Atreya passed it on to his students and they, including Jivaka, the Buddha's personal physician and patron saint of Tibetan medicine, taught and propagated it.

Now just as in the past time cycle the Buddha Kasyapa had taught medicine and those teachings had come into our time cycle in the lineage just described, so the Buddha Shakyamuni taught medicine in our present time cycle.

Tradition holds that the Buddha taught different medical works. Most important in terms of the medical tradition of Tibet is the mystical transformation during which the Buddha took on the form of the Medicine Buddha Vaidurya and gave the medical teaching which has come down to us as the *Gyu-zhi* (Tib. *rGyud-bzhi*), *The Four Tantras*, the most important text of Tibetan medicine. Its full title is *The Ambrosia Heart Tantra: The Secret Oral Teaching on the Eight Branches of the Science of Healing (bDud-rtsi snying-po yan-lag brgyad-pa gsang-ba man-ngag gi rgyud)*, but it is almost always referred to simply as the *Gyu-zhi*.

It was in the mystical medicine paradise called Tanatuk (Tib. *lTa-na-sdug*), literally "Pleasing When Looked Upon," that the Buddha, in the form of Vaidurya, expounded the teachings recorded as the *Gyu-zhi*. According to scriptures, saying that all people who want to meditate and reach nirvana and who want health, long life, and happiness should learn the science of medicine, the Medicine Buddha at Tanatuk projected two emanations. The first was an emanation of the Medicine Buddha's mind in the form of the sage Rigpai Yeshe (Tib. *Rig-pa'i ye-shes*). The second was an emanation of the Medicine Buddha's speech in the form of the sage Yilay Kye (Tib. *Yid-las-skyes*).

The whole medical teaching on the cause and treatment of disease that comprises the *Gyu-zhi* is recorded in the form of a dialogue between the emanations Rigpai Yeshe and Yilay Kye.

Attending the teaching in the medicine paradise were various gods, rishis, Buddhists, and non-Buddhists. They listened to the teaching and understood it in ways commensurate with their own knowledge and capacity. According to their comprehension, they wrote various medical treatises on what they had heard. Only Yilay Kye understood it completely. It is said that he wrote it down in 5,900 verses with lapis lazuli ink on sheets of pure gold, and that the dakinis keep it in their palace in Uddiyana.

The medicine paradise of Tanatuk is a Buddha-field, a pure land, a place beyond the illusion of subject and object. It is a mandala, a cosmogram, that specifically depicts the radiation of the sacred faculty of healing power, a faculty that is an inseparable part of all-embracing Buddha-nature.

The medicine mandala is particularly interesting because, traditionally, there are three different levels on which it exists: the outer, inner, and secret levels. The description of it contains the seed form of Buddhist medical mythology as well as the seed form of Ayurvedic herbal therapy.

In terms of its mystical external location, it is said to be Mount Meru, the sacred mountian in the center of the mandala that pictures our universe. In terms of more relative physicality, it is identified as being in Bodh Gaya, where the Buddha attained enlightenment, or in Uddiyana (north-west India or Afghanistan), where Buddhist tantra arose.

Shakyamuni Buddha as the Medicine Buddha Vaidurya is at the center of the mandala "Pleasing When Looked Upon." He resides in the middle of a celestial city in a transparent crystal palace where he is enthroned on a seat of lapis lazuli—the gem which is emblematic of medicine in Buddhism (Vaidurya's name means lapis lazuli).

Rays of healing light that ease all suffering shine forth from his luminous body. He is deep blue in color and sits in the full-lotus meditative posture. His left hand resting on his lap holds a begging bowl and his right hand, extended forward the gesture of giving, holds the "great medicine," myrobalan. He is radiant with the thirty-two marks of perfection and the eighty signs of great beauty which characterize all Buddhas. He is surrounded by attendant gods, rishis, Brahmins, Buddhists, non-Buddhists, the goddesses of medicine, the protectors of medicine, the three Great Protectors (Manjushri, Avalokitesvara, Vajrapani), his two closest disciples—Ananda and Shariputra, and the holders of the medicine lineage.

Sixteen thousand pillars made of the "five kinds of divine jewels" support the crystal palace. Inside it are also the three kinds of gems (of gods, bodhisattvas, and humans) that have healing powers.

All this is surrounded by arched balustrades, platforms for the offering goddesses, plus the five walls, eight steps and four gates of traditional mandala structure. The enchanting garden that surrounds the palace is populated with peaceful animals—pheasants, parrots, ducks, elephants, bears, peacocks—and filled with the sweet and healing scents of medicinal trees, incenses and perfumes.

In the four directions outside this celestial city where Vaidurya resides there are four medicine mountains that represent the seed of the whole herbal and Ayurvedic therapy. In the southern mountain grow the cures of all cold diseases; in the north, the cures of all fevers; in the west, all things that maintain good health; and in the east, the forests of myrobalan which cures every type of sickness.

It is said in the *Gyu-zhi* and elsewhere that not only does the medicine mandala exist as external, internal, and secret reality, but also that it should be practiced unto realization on these three levels. This means offering the mandala—devotion to the Medicine Buddha and the practice of medicine (external level); the practice of identifying oneself with the Medicine Buddha and one's world with the energies of the pure medicine land (inner level); and, the ultimate realization of the Buddha-nature as one's true nature, of oneself as the Medicine Buddha and one's own body as the medicine mandala (secret level). To practice the mandala in the last way is to realize the tri-kaya, the Buddha-nature of body, speech, and mind in oneself.

Among the fivefold division of Buddha-nature into the mandala of the Dhyani Buddhas, the prototypic Buddha of Medicine lives in the Eastern Buddha-field. Thus the Medicine Buddha is identified with Akshobhya, the Dhyani Buddha of the Eastern direction who is also blue in color.

The medicine mandala of the Eastern Buddha-field is also expressed, and many iconographical representations of it appear this way, as a circle of the eight Medicine Buddhas[35] that includes Sangye Menla, the Tibetan name of Vaidurya, and Shakyamuni, with the latter mainly at the center. Tara, Manjushri, and Vajrapani, all of whom have special healing manifestations, are usually in attendance.

Astrologically, the day of the Medicine Buddha is the eighth day of the lunar month. At that time the power of the Medicine Buddha and the healing deities is said to be especially strong, and this is when rituals for healing and for making medicines are performed.

Among the medicine deities, the female manifestation of the healing aspect of Buddha-nature has many forms. Besides Tara, there is the goddess Parnashabari, who is particularly known as the "Patroness of the Sick," destroyer of all diseases, epidemics, and undesirable spirits. She herself has eight forms and in most of them she is clad in medicine leaves. Other Buddhist goddesses associated with healing include Janguli, Mahachina, and Ekajati.

There are eight specific goddesses of medicine,[36] among them Dudtsi Ma (Tib. *bDud-rtsi-ma*), literally "the Nectar Mother."

According to Tibetan legendary history, one human incarnation of Dudtsi Ma was an Indian innkeeper's daughter named Yitogma

(Tib. *Yid-phrog-ma*). She was an extraordinarily beautiful and powerful creature credited with planting the medicine herbs and trees in and around Bodh Gaya, that is to say, the external manifest aspect of the medicine mandala. She consorted with siddhas, bodhisattvas, and kings, and her children furthered the medicine teaching. The most famous doctor-saint of Tibet, the Turquoise Physician, Yuthog, is said to be descended from her on one side and from Buddha's Shakya clan on the other.

Dudtsi Ma's wrathful archaic form is Dorje Phagmo (Tib. *rDo-rje phag-mo*), Vajravarahi, the "Diamond Sow-Headed Mother." She is the consort of the wrathful form of the Medicine Buddha, which is his aspect for driving away the evil spirits of disease: the Black Horse-Headed One, Tamdrin (*rTam-grin nag-po*). He is smokey colored. surrounded by flames and holds tantric weapons for subduing negative forces. The Black Horse-Headed One and the Diamond Sow-Headed Mother are pictured in sexual embrace. They represent the union of wisdom and skillful means, and from the power of their mantra hot molten metal flows into the chest of their enemies, subduing the demons of disease and transforming them into the Buddha-nature.

In addition to the Medicine Buddha Vaidurya and to the other medicine deities and goddesses, there is a special healing form of Padmasambhava, the "Lotus Born Guru," who established Tibetan Buddhism in Tibet. In his tantric form as the Medicine Buddha he is called Urgyen Menla.

Padmasambhava also has twelve separate manifestations and each of these has its own healing quality. For example, in his manifestation as the Great Guru of Great Bliss, Mahaguru Dewache, he is able to heal mental depression and psychological problems. In his form as Lodan Chogsed he can overcome problems of memory loss and can increase and sharpen intellectual powers of mind.

Tibet Seeks the Medical Learning of the World

As we have already described, Tibetan medical knowledge is based primarily on Indian Ayurveda. The connection between Buddhism and Ayurveda was vital. The history of the establishment of Buddhism in Tibet is also the history of the establishment of Ayurvedic and tantric medicine there.

But there were other important transcultural influences on Tibetan medicine. From Chinese medicine came the systems of pulse diagnosis, measurement and inspection of the tongue, and acupuncture. The advanced Persian medical system, which incorporated the ancient Greek medical system, also had some influence on the Tibetan system. The Tibetans took the best of these teachings and added them to Ayurvedic, Buddhist, and tantric medicine adopted from India. They also added urine analysis, their major indigenous contribution to Ayurvedic medical science; a good Tibetan doctor could diagnose and prescribe a cure simply by urine analysis.

Tibet had a reputation as a land of medicine herbs in pre-Buddhist times. There was a "Palace of Medicine Herbs" in the Yarlung Valley where the early Tibetan kingdom first acquired its sense of itself as a distinct nation and culture. The marvelous quality of Tibetan healing herbs was known in ancient China, and mention of them found its way into early Chinese pharmacological texts.

The indigenous shamanic religious culture called Bon had its own medical tradition. The Bon-pos knew the magical and medical properties of the wealth of herbs growing on their sub-Himalayan plateaus. But the systematized science of medicine in pre-Buddhist Tibet was limited, and Bon medical texts, which were written after the importation of Buddhism, are said to show the influence of Ayurveda.

It appears that Indian Ayurvedic knowledge spread to Tibet around the fifth century when the first influences of Buddhism also began to be felt there. At that time Tibet was still without a written language, but the medical knowledge from abroad was absorbed in a limited fashion into the native Tibetan healing culture. Unlike the situation with Indian Buddha-Dharma, there was no resistance to taking on a foreign medical teaching. Indeed, it is recorded that the Tibetan kings showed a keen interest in it.[37]

The first Indian Buddhists to bring Ayurveda to Tibet were two fifth century physician-saints, a man named Vijay and a woman named Belha. The goddess Tara had appeared to them in a vision urging them to go there, and so they went to Tibet to spread the medical teaching. Their work greatly pleased the Tibetan king, Lhatho Thori Nyantsen, who awarded them many honors at court and requested them to remain in his land in order to establish the Ayurvedic tradition. Therefore Vijay married and his son, Dungi Thorchog, was trained by both Vijay and Belha. Dungi Thorchog is celebrated as Tibet's first native lama-doctor, and his heirs, too, carried on the medical vocation. This manner of passing knowledge through a family lineage is a major way medical teachings were preserved in Tibet.

King Srongtsan Gampo (Tib. *Srong-btsan sGam-po*) formally introduced Buddhism to Tibet during the first half of the seventh century. At that time Tibet was beginning a two hundred year reign as a major power in Central Asia and was surrounded by Buddhist countries—China, India, Nepal, Kashmir, and Afghanistan—at the high point of their development of Mahayana and tantric Buddhist traditions.

King Srongtsan Gampo converted to Buddhism, probably due to the influence of his two Buddhist wives, one from China and one from Nepal. The King began to send messengers to India, Nepal, and China to gather Buddhist books and teachings, including those on medicine, and these were brought to Tibet.

In order to translate the Sanskrit and Pali texts he was gathering from all over the Buddhist world, the King directed that an alphabet be derived from the Sanskrit Devanagari script. Previous to this development there was no written Tibetan language. The new Tibetan script made it possible to translate faithfully and exactly the Sanskrit and Pali Buddhist texts. The translation that began then and went on for centuries was so perfect and systematic that today lost Indian works are being translated from Tibetan back into their original languages.

In particular pursuit of medical knowledge, King Srongtsan Gampo held the first international medical conference in Tibet. Doctors came from India, Persia, and China. Each one translated one of his native medical works into Tibetan and presented it to the King. They also composed a new medical treatise through a joint endeavor. The visiting Persian doctor, Galenos,[38] was asked to remain in Tibet as the court physician. He married and had three sons, all of whom began separate medical family lineages.

While medical knowledge increased steadily after Srongtsan Gampo's reign, the Buddha Dharma did not spread beyond a limited following in the royal court. Some of the succeeding kings were strongly against Buddhism and actively sought its demise.

It was during the reign of King Trison Detsen (Tib. *Khri-srong-lde-btsan*) that the Dharma really began to prosper in Tibet. To establish Dharma in his land, the king first invited the distinguished Bengali Abbot Shantarakshita to come and teach. The reserved and gentle abbot, a great scholar and monk, found the Tibetan people too wild, unsuited to his style of teaching. He suggested to the young king that he invite the Indian tantric saint Padmasambhava to come to

subdue the demons and the devil-worshippers, to establish the
Dharma, and build Tibet's first monastery.

In 749 Padmasambhava accepted the King's invitation, went to
Tibet, subdued the negative forces, and so firmly established the
Dharma there that from that time on Vajrayana Buddhism and all the

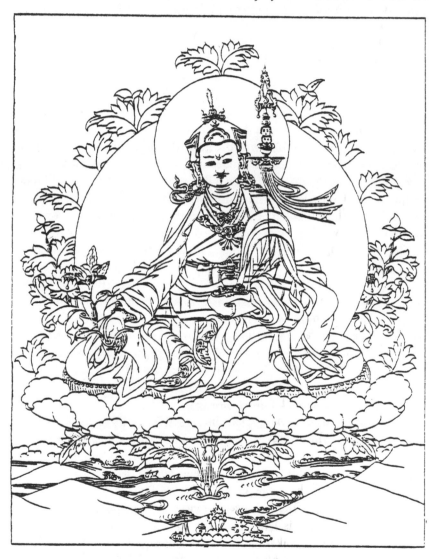

Figure 10 Urgyen Menla, Guru Padmasambhava in his healing aspect holding the
"all-conquering" myrobalan plant. Padmasambhava studied and mastered Ayurvedic and siddha medicine in India, receiving the "Life-Saving Essence of
Medicine." He gave many kinds of medicine teachings in Tibet.

sciences it included became the one and only consuming interest, life-focus, and belief of the Tibetan people. From that time on Tibetan Buddhism and Tibetan culture were inseparable.

It is possible to imagine the critical situation which a great realized being like Padmasambhava saw Buddhism to be in at that time, and thus to recognize how urgent was the need to establish the entire Buddhist lineage in a protected stronghold like Tibet. For although Buddhism was still reaching new heights of spiritual and artistic development in the Indian lands, the political order had begun to crumble. The reigns of the great Dharma kings like Ashoka and later the Indo-Scythian ruler Kanishka were long over. In Padmasambhava's own land of Uddiyana where tantra had arisen and in other north-west lands like Gandhara the invading barbarian Huns had already devastated Buddhist sanctuaries, shrines, civilizations, and art. Where hundreds of thousands of shrines, temples, and monasteries had stood in Swat, most were deserted and desecrated by the 7th century. Buddhism was no longer expanding in India, political stability was on the wane, and signs of future dark times were there for enlightened ones to read.

Padmasambhava is known to Tibetans as the "Second Buddha." Shakyamuni Buddha is said to have prophesized his birth and that he would reveal the inner and esoteric meanings of the Dharma. According to Tibetan belief, Padmasambhava, or "Guru Rinpoche," was miraculously born on a lotus and is the Nirmanakaya aspect of the Buddha Amitabha.

Padmasambhava is a historical figure who was renowned for his mastery of all the tantric practices. He propogated the tantric teachings because only they would be appropriate for beings in the dark and degenerate age of materialism.

Padmasambhava was also a great master of tantric medicine. He composed medical works like the *Nectar Essence* (Tib. *bDud-rtsi'i snying-po*) that were preserved in Tibet. More essentially, he gave many different kinds of medical teachings, including prophesies about new diseases that would manifest in the future and the prescriptions and meditations to cure and prevent them. To benefit future beings he hid these texts in various places and ways so that they would be discovered when needed. All his hidden teachings are called terma (Tib. *gter-ma*) and form a special body of literature within the Nyingmapa tradition. In addition to special medical teachings most of Guru Rinpoche's termas, which cover a whole range of tantric meditational practices and sadhanas, contain some medical instructions, i.e., how to use the sadhana for healing purposes and directions for making specific medicines.

Padmasambhava established the Dharma, built Tibet's first monastery, Samye (created in the form of a mandala, including an image of Sangye Menla), initiated the king and others into his lineage of esoteric Buddhism, and prophesized that in future times, after centuries of unbroken lineage in Tibet, the Dharma would go to the West.

Guru Rinpoche, King Trison Detsen, and Abbot Shantarakshita form a trinity of the early Tibetan tantrayana, as do Guru Rinpoche's three major disciples—Guru Rinpoche's consort Yeshe Tsogyal, King Trison Detsen, and the translator Vairochana. Most carefully they all nurtured the diamond-seed of Dharma.

Padmasambhava and Abbot Shantarakshita oversaw the education of Vairochana, who became Tibet's first great translator. They sent him to India to receive teachings. Vairochana met numerous Indian pandits and siddhas and received instruction and initiations from them. Again, as has been emphasized, there was no distinction between religious and medical teachings. It was all part of the Dharma. So, in addition to the important religious texts which Vairochana procured, translated, and mastered, there was also the medical work that became the most crucial in Tibetan medical literature, the *Gyu-zhi*. Vairochana received the teaching of the *Gyu-zhi* from Ashvaghosha's disciple, Chandranandana.

On Vairochana's return to Tibet he met Yuthog Yontan Gonpo (*gYu-thog yon-tan mgon-po*), Tibet's first great doctor-saint. Vairochana gave the *Gyu-zhi* teaching to Yuthog, then, according to Padmasambhava's prophetic direction, the book was hidden in a pillar of Samye Monastery until a future time when Padmasambhava said it would be discovered when people were ready to understand it. In fact, the *Gyu-zhi* was extracted from its hiding place by Trapa Ngonshe (*Grva-pa mngon-shes*) in 1038.[39] Because the *Gyu-zhi* was a hidden then rediscovered work it can be classified as a terma.

King Trison Detsen so valued the Tibetan medical tradition and all medicine systems that he decided to hold a debate among the greatest doctors in Asia to examine each tradition's best points. He invited doctors from India, China, Kashmir, Persia, Nepal, Mongolia, Sinkiang, and Afghanistan. Yuthog Yontan Gonpo represented Tibet. All translated texts from their own systems and presented them to the King. The doctor from China became the King's court physician and started his own family medical lineage in Tibet, which was called

"Foreign Doctors." But, according to Tibetan history, it was the Tibetan doctor Yuthog who won the debate.

Yuthog Yontan Gonpo, or the "Turquoise Roof Physician," is a prime example of the lama-doctors and physician-saints of Tibet, an exalted and holy model of the healer drawn from the example of the Medicine Buddha himself.

Yuthog was an ordained monk until the age of eighty when he married to propagate the lineage. An accomplished siddha who could perform psychic feats of miraculous power, Yuthog lived to be 125 years old. He is believed by Tibetans to be an emanation of the speech of the Medicine Buddha.

Under the force of Yuthog's brilliant medical learning, his peerless devotion to medical science, and his spiritual attainments, the Tibetan medical system was advanced and compiled into texts and treatises that unified the knowledge of diagnosis and treatment. Yuthog visited India three times to compare the Tibetan and Indian systems, going to centers of Buddhist learning like Nalanda to receive new teachings. He wrote supplements to the *Gyu-zhi* and many other texts.

The period from Yuthog's life in the eighth century to that of his namesake and descendent in the twelfth century is considered by some as the "golden age" of Tibetan medicine. During that time more medical knowledge continued to be acquired from foreign sources, most especially India, as part of the enormous body of Buddhist literature the Tibetans so dedicatedly and one-pointedly sought out, and Tibetan medicine flourished.

Tibet's second great translator and religious founder, Rinchen Zangpo, lived during that time. He spent over ten years in India acquiring teachings and initiations. From a Kashmiri pandit he learned Ashvaghosha's medical work, *The Collection of the Essence of the Eight Branches,* Chandranandana's commentary on it, and many other medical treatises. He passed these teachings on to his own Tibetan disciples, who in turn wrote new medical works.

The second Yuthog, the twelfth century namesake of the earlier Tibetan physician, received the teachings of the *Gyu-zhi* which had been extracted from its hiding place at Samye Monastery. His religious knowledge was extensive, but he especially emphasized medicine. He went to India six times for teachings, and went to Ceylon to learn their version of the *Gyu-zhi.* He produced a new version of the *Gyu-zhi.* In addition, he wrote an exhaustive commentary on it called *The Eighteen Auxiliary Aids,* which was in part an introduction to the history of medicine. By mastering the teaching of the *Gyu-zhi*, he was able to spread its teaching throughout Tibet. It seems his edition of the *Gyu-zhi* has remained the standard version.

Actually, it is almost impossible to determine the exact authorship of the *Gyu-zhi*, and there are variations on its history. But, in short, most agree that it was transmitted by Shakyamuni in the form of the Medicine Buddha via two emanations he projected from a state of deep meditation. Jivaka was among those who received the teaching, and it was passed down through a lineage of Buddhist physician-saints to Chandranandana, who gave a written version of it to the Tibetan Vairochana.

Vairochana translated it in the eighth century and presented it to the Tibetan king, Trison Detsen, and his court physician, the first Yuthog. Padmasambhava subsequently hid it in Samye Monastery, where it remained until the middle of the eleventh century when it was taken out by Trapa Ngonshe, who gave it to Khuton Tarmatra, who, in turn, gave it to the second Yuthog. The second Yuthog mastered it and apparently redacted it. Just how much it was revised (if at all) then or at any point is hard to measure since the Sanskirt original no longer exists. Parts of the present *Gyu-zhi*, however, do contain elements which were most likely not in the Indian version— mention of uniquely Tibetan foods, plants unknown in India, Mongolian cauterization, Chinese pulse theory, etc. The original eighth century Tibetan translation, having been replaced in a pillar of Samye Monastery by its discoverer, was supposedly still there as recently as twenty years ago.

By the 13th century the Moslems had swept over the Indian regions and utterly destroyed all traces of Buddhist religion, culture and learning, putting monks to the sword and throwing texts to the winds. This meant two things: first, Tibetans could no longer go to India for teachings, but this was not so important since they had already brought almost all the spiritual and scientific lineages back to Tibet as living initiated lineages. And second, this left Tibet preserving the whole canon of Mahayana and Tantrayana Sanskrit texts, including those on medicine, a great many of which were lost or destroyed in India.

The Tibetan religious canon is divided into two sections, the Kanjur, the words of the Buddha, and the Tanjur, other texts and treatises. There are about twenty-one Ayurvedic works that were translated and incorporated into the Tanjur, some of which according to the foremost scholar of Indo-Tibetan Ayurveda, Dr. Bhagwan

Dash, are lost in the original Sanskrit. Still others are completely unknown to the Indian Ayurvedic world.[40]

Further, says Bhagwan Dash, *Gyu-zhi,* a medical work not included in the religious canon, shows a significant advancement of medical knowledge beyond the literature of the classical Ayurvedic tradition that exists today in India. For example, he notes that embryology in the *Gyu-zhi* is described in terms of weekly stages but in existent Ayurveda it is only known in terms of months.

Ayurvedic tradition declined because of internal political and cultural conflicts in India and because the real meaning of siddha medicine (Ayurvedic alchemy or tantric essence healing) began to get lost. Also surgery, so famous as Indian Ayurveda's great contribution in the history of medicine, had completely declined. The Moslem invasion caused breaks in the tradition and loss of texts. It also brought its own medical system, Yunani, and this mixed with the Indian one. Centuries later, the British empire in India had a similar effect, breaking tradition and introducing modern medicine which mixed with the existing strains of Ayurveda and Yunani. Ironically, it was the influence of British orientalists that caused the revival of classical Ayurveda, as well as the revival of interest in Indian esoteric traditions of self-knowledge. Although Ayurvedic medicine still participates in the health care system of modern India, it is different from the classical tradition, much of it having been well mixed and developed with the Islamic system.[41] Nevertheless, it should be made clear that Ayurveda has survived for millenniums in India and continues to be practiced extensively there.

Tibetan Medicine on Its Own

In the 14th century there were two famous Tibetan doctors, Jangpa (Tib. *Byang-pa*) and Zurkarpa (Tib. *Zur-mkar-pa*), who wrote and taught exhaustively. Both Jangpa and Zurkarpa had rival medical systems named after them. Each of these two doctors wrote one of the three main commentaries on the *Gyu-zhi.* The two systems continued without interruption, but by the 17th century there was some decline. Therefore the Fifth Dalai Lama decided to institute Tibet's first medical school.

Initially the school was at Drepung Monastery, but then the Dalai Lama and his Regent, after choosing a spot by mystical means, built a school-hospital monastic complex called the Iron Mountain or Chagpori, so named for the rockhill in Lhasa on which it

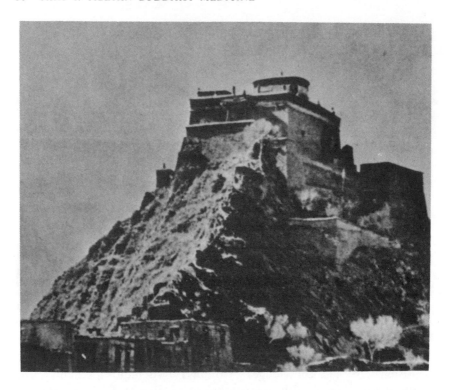

Figure 11 Chagpori Medical College, built in the 17th century by Desi Sangye Gyatso, the Regent who ruled Tibet for many years after the death of the Fifth Dalai Lama; he was an outstanding scholar who wrote many important medical treatises. The building was destroyed by the Chinese Army in 1959.

was built. It became the spiritual center for medicine in Tibet, known throughout surrounding countries as a place of medical learning and secret herbal cures made by the lama-doctors.

Mongolian doctors and medical students used to make pilgrimages to Chagpori as they had, centuries before and especially after the conversion of Kublai Khan to the Dharma, taken up Tibetan Ayurveda with great enthusiasm, translating the major medical works into Mongolian and adopting the whole medical tradition. (Mongolian Ayurveda, which is really Tibetan Buddhist medicine, survives to this day in the USSR.)[42]

Sangye Gyatso, the Regent of the Fifth Dalai Lama and the most politically powerful person in the Tibet of his time, was also an accomplished physician. He knew and practiced both the *Zur-lugs* and *Byang-lugs* medical systems. And he wrote the third and most important commentary on the *Gyu-zhi,* the *Blue Lapis Lazuli (Vaidurya sngon-po).*

After Chagpori was established, the Regent declared that every main monastery would henceforth have a lama-doctor from there. This was the beginning of "public health" in Tibet. It must be mentioned, however, that in spite of their medical system, the majority of Tibetans were, on the whole, inclined to persist in highly unsanitary habits due, in part, to the high altitude and cold, to primitive living conditions, and lack of education among the common people.

Tibetan medicine was famed throughout Central Asia, especially the skill of the lama-doctors with urine analysis and herbal medications. And even more renowned were the Dharma medicines that the lamas produced with their yogic and mystical powers. The techniques and ingredients of these medicines were scrupulously concealed from exploiters and the merely curious.

There is a story recorded in *Manchu Anatomy,* written by a Western missionary in China during the 17th century, about how Emperor K'ang Hsi liked to have competitions between rival medical systems (as the early Tibetan kings did as well). One missionary-surgeon had suffered acute colic while on the north-west frontier with the Emperor. No Western or Chinese doctor could cure him, and upon learning this the Emperor demanded that they write up their diagnosis and treatment as a sort of test. Then he called in a Tibetan lama-doctor who "cured the patient in half an hour with a voluminous suppository made on the spot with oil, wax, tow and herbal powders."[43]

A measure of the high regard with which physicians were held in Tibet is shown in the title accorded to the greatest ones among them: "King of the Gods," the "All Knowing One," the latter an epithet reserved for bodhisattvas. Ideally, a doctor was expected to practice compassion at all times and equally towards all beings, to perfect his skill for their sake, and to always remember that a physician was a representative of the Medicine Buddha and the holy lineage of medicine teaching.

In this ideal there is no separation of healing skill from Dharma. The greater a person's heart-realization of true Dharma, the greater a doctor he can be, for he will have the two-fold Buddha-nature aspects of wisdom and compassion, rendering him more capable of understanding the depths of the medical science and serving the physical, emotional and spiritual needs of his patients. He is responsible for providing the spiritual and emotional support crucial for physical and, in the case of psychiatry, mental cure. His ability to be skillfully supportive to his patients is an outcome of the wisdom and compassion developed with Buddhist training. It would be hard to find a higher model for a doctor to follow than the selfless, skillful healing power of enlightened being represented by Bhaishajyaguru, the Medicine Buddha.

This is, of course, the ideal level. No doubt not all Tibetan doctors and lama-doctors measured up to it, but many did. The greatest doctors of Tibet were also great lamas, beings whose philosophical wisdom and depth of meditation went way beyond the limits of any secular concept of medicine and medical morality.

This was not simply true of a prototypical lama doctor like the "Turquoise Physician," Yuthog, who lived so long ago, who propagated the medicine teachings, who practiced medicine with extreme genius, and who accomplished the ultimate Dharma medicine by transmuting his physical body into rainbow light at the time of his death. There has consistently been a stream of great lamas, yogis, and saints who turned their wisdom and powers of mind to the subject of medicine. And this tradition has continued to the present.

In the late 19th and early 20th century, Lama Mipham continued this tradition. The most renowned scholar of his time, Lama Mipham systematized the sutras and philosophical tantras and wrote thirty-two volumes including works on music, logic, astrology, alchemy, and medicine. He compiled and practiced hundreds of ritual meditations of various Buddhas, and he did a seven year retreat. His numerous medical writings include an area called "secret healing" (sman-ngang) which combines tantric and somatic medical practices with Dharma. He also wrote a text on the healing properties of gems, a text on the medicinal uses of five Tibetan grasses, and a commentary on the major points of the Gyu-zhi.

Another great lama of the late 19th century who was also a great doctor was Jamgon Kongtrul, a founder of Tibet's ecumenical "ri-mé" movement and guru to the 15th Gyalwa Karmapa. His medical writings include a practical medical handbook that is still used by contemporary Tibetan physicians.

In the beginning of the 20th century, during the time of the 13th Dalai Lama, the outstanding physician-lama Khyenrab Norbu built a new medical college in Lhasa called the House of Medicine and Astronomy. He was a child prodigy when, at a young age, he became a monk. He began studying medicine at fourteen and within two years had memorized the entire *Gyu-zhi* (Tibetan doctors were expected to commit it to memory) and within four more years he understood the entire teaching and passed his medical examinations without a flaw. At the age of thirty-three he started building the new medical school.

Students at both of Tibet's medical colleges followed a rigorous routine combining prayer and religious studies (beginning at 3 A.M. with a prayer to the Bodhisattva of Wisdom, Manjushri) with the study of the arts and sciences and all the special medical studies. They went on special outings to identify and collect medical plants and to be examined on their knowledge of them. Strict general examinations were held each year. It took six years to complete the entire course.

Qualifying exams for the medical schools were extremely arduous, and a fourteen year course of fundamental studies was usually required before starting. Generally, it was said to take thirty years to master medicine.

Rechung Rinpoche says in his book *Tibetan Medicine* that the College of Medicine and Astronomy held a daily clinic and treated people for free. He says further that:

> The country districts had their own doctors sent there by the government in order to look after the sick. There were also many private doctors who charged for their services but never asked for a definite price to be paid for a medicine. It was left to the patient to pay as much as he wanted or could pay. Private doctors, too, would never take a fee from poor patients and would treat them for nothing.[44]

David Snellgrove and Hugh Richardson, in their book *A Cultural History of Tibet,* take a rather different view of the medical services available in Tibet. They say that the monks at the medical colleges did not especially go out into the villages to cure the sick, but rather stayed at the medical monasteries making medicants and herbal pills and taking money for their treatments, and that, in any case, the people of Tibet put more faith in charms and amulets than in medicine.

Nevertheless, then Snellgrove and Richardson go on to say that they had some Tibetan medicine and it worked quite well, and that "there is no doubt that some Tibetans possess a great deal of practical knowledge" and that "Tibetan medical practice is a study which merits serious attention" and, finally, that it should be dealt with on an empirical basis of testing the cures and medications.[45]

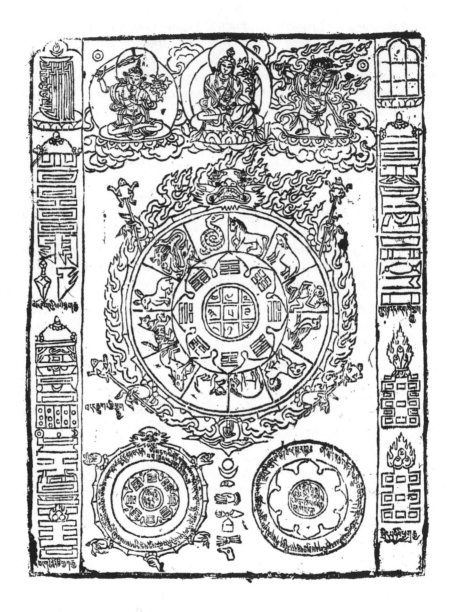

Figure 12 An astrological chart based on the astrological system set forth in the Kalachakra Tantra. Astrology is an integral part of Tibetan medicine, and Tibetan doctors must master it in order to diagnose and treat disease. For example, different types of illness, pulse beats, humoral influences, etc., are prevalent during different astrological periods.

5

Tantric Medicine

The tantric medicine of Tibet provides the bridge between the religious medicine of Dharma and the rational or scientific medical system.

Tantra is the mysticism of direct sacred knowledge, the gnosis of absolute truth discovered on the relative plane through uniting the polarized energies of the human body and on the absolute plane by direct realization of the primordial Buddha-nature.

In Buddhist tantric yoga the sacred universe is internalized. The basic practice is to understand the correspondences between "the cruder karmic body," the human body, and the body of absolute truth, "the pure essence of Buddha's Body," which has been concealed by clingings and confusions. The intermediary links between these two bodies are the subtle life-force airs, psychic veins, and vital essences which support physical existence. Through tantric practice, the clingings and confusions are cleared away and these life-forces, veins, and essences are purified and transformed to reveal the three inherent bodies of Buddhahood. Garma C.C. Chang has said that tantrism is "the view of the unity of identity of Samsara and Nirvana, sublimation of Passion-Desires, and unfoldment of the Innate Trikaya."[46]

Throughout Buddhism, but especially in its tantric forms, a three-dimensional structuring of reality—the Three Jewels, the Three Roots, the Three Kayas—expresses three inseparable but distinct levels of one reality: outer, inner, and secret; exoteric, esoteric and absolute; the trinity of Buddha-nature.

The expression of absolute truth as the three-fold Buddha body is the doctrinal foundation of tantric practice and tantric medicine; it is also the template of our actual embodied existence with its three aspects—mental, subtle (vital) and physical—and for the three kinds of Tibetan medicine—Dharmic, tantric, and somatic—which affect those three aspects.

The overall picture of Tibetan medicine is similarly complex in this way, an interwoven expression of non-linear, triadic relationships linking the spiritual, psychic, and physical life of the individual and the universe. In Buddhist tantric medicine, that entire universe is seen to be within the individual. Tantric medicine deals with the vital psycho-physical energies of the internalized universe as a means of transforming it and the outer universe. The subtle psycho-physical energies generate the physical body much in the same way that they themselves have been generated by the formless processes of mind.

This energetic-essence body is called the "subtle body" (Tib. *phra-bai lus*), rather a suitable term since it embraces the invisible yet underlying forces of life. Tantric practices aim at purifying the components of the subtle body as a means of realizing the three-fold Buddha body.

Tantric medicine is the "inner" level of medicine, between the "secret" Dharma medicine, which is the medicine of religion and the direct perception of absolute truth, and the "outer" medicine, which is the medicine of the somatic body in the physical universe. These are the three bodies of medicine, and like the actual tri-kaya they are distinct but inseparable.

The vast, qualityless, unborn and undying pure reality, "That-ness," is called the Dharmakaya ("wisdom body," corresponding to Buddha mind). It is realized by transforming ordinary awareness to supreme awareness of the all-embracing void. The reality of subtle manifestations such as light and energy, sounds, colors, etc. is known as Sambhogakaya ("enjoyment body," corresponding to Buddha speech). It is the purified form of the "subtle body" upon which the tantric processes to be discussed here work. The Nirmanakaya (the "manifestation body," Buddha body) is the physical body in its purified or realized state. These three kayas represent the levels on which the Buddha-essence is inherent in all sentient life; but it is obscured and unrecognized. Realization of the Buddha-essence, Buddhahood, is the ultimate goal of Tibetan Buddhism and Tibetan medicine. The three levels of Tibetan medicine—Dharmic, tantric and somatic—correspond to the three kayas: absolute reality, radiant clarity, and unobstructed action.

It is a basic of the Tibetan system that religion and medicine are never really separate and this is what provides it with such an all-encompassing definition of health. But for practical purposes, religion and medicine form separate disciplines. In between these two are the healing process of Buddhist tantricism. The art of knowing and using these forces in relation to spiritual development is called tantric yoga; in relation to health we may call it tantric healing.

Through the practice of tantra and the realization of Buddha-nature (expressed as the tri-kaya) various miraculous, supernatural powers arise and, in terms of tantric medicine, these are related to healing power. For example, among the "Eight Siddhis" or powers that arise as "the mundane accomplishment" of tantric practice is "the attainment of magical pills with miraculous powers of healing."[47] The "transcendental accomplishment" is the realization of the three kayas.

Mystical or psychic powers, siddhis, arise naturally as one progresses on the path, not only in the tantric tradition. Lord Buddha himself described the five "higher" kinds of awareness that are possessed by ordinary beings, although few of us are able to realize them. One of these is "miraculous power"; others are the recollection of former lives and knowing others' thoughts.

When the tantric processes are understood, it becomes clear that they are not some religious "hocus-pocus" by which we delude ourselves and others. These tantric processes are the skillful manipulation of psycho-physical energies by beings who, through the practice of Dharma, especially meditation, have refined their introspective mental abilities to such a point that they can perceive the otherwise invisible aspects of manifest being, much in the same way that a microscope is a refined extension of human sight, whose power is vastly enlarged. The vision of the spiritually and yogically advanced adept is sometimes called the "wisdom-eye." Among other things, it can perceive solid form in terms of its essential and subtle density and luminosity—like seeing the aura and color of energy, like seeing with X-ray or ultra-sound vision instead of with the naked eye.

Tantric processes are similarly real, not incomprehensible miracles. But they are, especially in Tibetan Buddhism, concealed in symbolic terms of a religious culture which we do not, as scientific modern Westerners, readily understand or relate to. And therefore they seem alien, bewildering and superstitious. Yet the cryptic coding and concealed meaning of the symbolic language of tantra was intentional. It was done in order to keep the unworthy and uninitiated "in the dark."

Fortunately, much has been done in the past decade and a half to reveal the functional basis of tantra and to clear away the veil of other-worldliness (and therefore the presumed irrelevance) that has surrounded it. It is a highly sophisticated and complex system, a sort of para-science of psychic and spiritual reality, and in terms of medicine, of psychic and spiritual healing.

Mystic Physiology:
The Psychic Channels, Airs, and Essences

Within the subtle body there are said to be numerous subtle psychic channels (Tib. *rtsa*), airs or forces (Tib. *rlung*), and essences (Tib. *thig-le*). These three are the main components of the subtle body and they provide the crucial link between the diamond vajra body and the substantive physical body.

Their interrelationship is stated as follows: The body depends on the psychic channels, the channels depend on the psychic forces or airs, and the psychic force depends on the mind. So emotions support the "lung" or psychic force, the psychic force supports the channels, and the channels support the body. The psychic force controls everything. It is like an "untamed wild horse." Mind rides on it and runs around without any control.

The subtle pathways support the vital airs which in turn support the mind, but the absolute mind-essence is spread throughout the body in the thigle essences. The yogic manipulation of the pathways, airs, and essences by breathing, visualization, mantra, and yogic exercises controls the forces of mind and body and clears a "direct path" to the realization of Buddhahood. Since the source of negative emotions, diseases, and "demons" is the mind, by pacifying and taming the mind, all the external negative forces and diseases can be pacified and brought to exhaustion.

The subtle veins correspond to but are not the same as the physical nerves and veins. When purified and controlled through tantra, they correspond to the Nirmanakaya. The subtle airs correspond to the bodily humoral airs which are defined in Tibetan medicine as being of five types; when purified they correspond to the Sambhogakaya. The subtle thigle essence corresponds to the physical semen, menstrual blood, and vital secretions; its purified form corresponds with the Dharmakaya.

The psychic nerves or mystic channels are numerous; they are sometimes numbered 72,000 but are also said to be uncountable.

However, there are three main channels: the central vein (Tib. *dbu-ma*); the right channel (Tib. *ro-ma*); and the left channel (Tib. *rkyang-ma*).

It is a measure of the non-concreteness of the subtle body that rather than being an exact system which is always described in the same way, these subtle veins and the chakras associated with them vary in description depending on the medical system or on the particular tantric system involved. They are not solid realities which one can point out like in the physical body, in spite of the fact that people often try to make exact identifications with particular parts of the body. Such identifications do not hold up. There are, however, more general correspondences which do have meaning and significance. In any case, the variations of their description points to the fact that the meditator or adept has to find them for himself, and to locate them according to his own yogic and meditative abilities and the particular spiritual practice or *sadhana* he is following. I will describe them here according to the system most generally used.

The central channel runs from the top of the head beneath the soft spot on the skull (the so-called "Gate of Brahma"), to a space located four fingerwidths beneath the navel. The channel represents the absolute aspect, consciousness, non-dual wisdom. The vein is straight, hollow, luminous and blue. It is said to be as thin as an arrow shaft. It is not the same as the spinal cord, but corresponds to it. It is the subtle verticle axis of the subtle body as the spine is the gross one.

The right column branches off from the central one just above the eyebrows and runs parallel to the central one, an inch or so away from it, rejoining it just above the lowest part of it below the navel. The left column does exactly the same thing on the other side of the body. This is the way it is visualized in meditation, but actually the two side columns intertwine with the central channel at various important points along it. (It should be noted that in some tantric systems, as well as in medicine, the central column is considered to extend all the way to the sexual organ.)

Both side veins are thinner than the central one, but are also hollow and luminous. The right one is red and represents the feminine aspect, blood, and, most importantly, the basic desire-grasping obscuration.

The left side is white. It represents the male aspect, the element water and the basic hatred-aversion obscuration. When the airs and essences in the three veins are consciously held together where the three join below the navel, then the mystic heat (Tib. *gtum-mo*) arises.

The subtle airs contain the life-force or *prana* (Tib. *srog-lung*). The Tibetans identify a reciprocal character between mind and the life-air, so that controlling and stabilizing the airs also stabilizes the mind. This is a basic principle of all yoga. We can understand this relationship if we think of how our breathing pattern alters depending on our mental and emotional state. We have only to think of the difference in our breathing when we are angry and when we are concentrating. Moods and feelings are reflected in the rhythm of the breath. Therefore, we can affect the mind and consciousness by manipulating the breath.

The two side columns inflate with the outer airs that are drawn in through the nostrils. Usually these airs disperse all over the body through the numerous pathways, and internally they are called the "karmic airs" because they carry the force of the mental obscurations. But a yogi controls these karmic airs and makes them join the central column. That is, he controls the force of karmic defilements and transmutes them by bringing them into the "middle path."

Thus it is said that an adept who controls his breath can transmute the three poisons into the the three wisdoms by control of these three pathways. Air is drawn in and circulated downward through the outer two veins. It joins the central column at its lowermost part. After holding the breath while the three are connected at the base of the central column, the essence of the "wisdom air" is kept in the central column, while the defilements and negative karmas are expelled with the exhalation.

The vital essences or "thigles" are of two types: absolute and relative. The relative thigles are of many kinds and pervade the body as vital essence-drops.

All the thigles in the body are generated from the main thigle in the central channel at the heart center. This central thigle is composed of the pure quintessence of the five elements (represented by orbs of five-colored light); it also contains the essence of the life-force. The red mother essence-drop and the white father essence-drop are generated from it and move downwards and upwards, respectively, in the central column.

All the thigles are within the hollows of the subtle channels and are the supports for life and awareness. When the negative emotions tangle the channels, this results in the blockage of energies or winds and consequently the thigles become more gross. When they are maintained in the body as gross essences rather than wisdom essences, the world outside is perceived negatively. Transmuting the thigles into their refined wisdom nature, the world is perceived in a positive way, and one's awareness blossoms as bliss and peace. Thus the purpose of tantric yoga is to untangle the knots in the channels, purify the karmic wind-energies, and reveal the thigles as the nature of wisdom.

The thigles are, through yogic practice, drawn into the hollows of the central column along with the airs. By controlling all the airs and essences and sending them into the central column, and further activating those essences within the central column with the force of the "mystic heat" one opens the mandalas of the chakras, the inner psychic centers along the central column, and sets a straight course to full enlightenment.

The absolute thigle is pervasive. It represents the Buddha-nature and exists within all the subtle pathways, airs, and essences. It is the "Great Thigle" which is the same as the absolute bodhi-mind. As it was said by Lama Mipham:

> Within the extraordinary veins, air and [thigle], which are the essence of the Vajra Body, and originating simultaneously with them from the beginning (like camphor and the smell of camphor) is the Great Thigle; it is self-illuminating, changeless, stainless, the Enlightened Mind, unpolluted, Great Bliss and self-arisen Primordial Wisdom.[48]

Realization of the great thigle is tantamount to enlightenment. This is the transformation that occurs when the subtle airs and essences are in the central column and become respectively the inherent wisdom-air (Tib. *ye-shes-kyi rlung*) and bodhi-mind.

Therefore, the central channel is the most important space within the subtle body; in its realized state it is called the "Wisdom Channel." When it is controlled and purified, it completely transforms the basic ignorance (which it represents) that is the cause of all delusion. It is the "Middle Vein" like the "Middle Way," and in this sense it indicates that its nature is shunyata and that it avoids the two extremes of nihilism and eternalism (the polarities of energies represented by the other two veins). This vein is not produced by visualization. It is discovered by visualization and meditation. It is always there. It is the main link between the purely spiritual and purely physical worlds. Realization of the karmic airs as the wisdom-air and the thigles as the bodhi-mind within this central channel at the heart center is equivalent to realization of the Dharmakaya.

Tantric mystic physiology of the subtle body is directly related to the somatic physiology of regular medicine, and the tantric practices of manipulating it bear directly on tantric healing. For example, the system of subtle veins and pathways are the channels used and manipulated in Tibetan acupuncture and moxibustion.

The three humors of air, bile and phlegm correspond to the subtle essences, energies and channels. Blockages on the subtle plane cause diseases on the physical or humoral plane, while purification of the subtle plane brings about realization of the spiritual bodies (kayas). The Dharmakaya is the purified air; the Sambhogakaya is the purified bile principle; and the Nirmanakaya is the purified phlegm.

The three central veins of tantric yoga are directly linked to the physical veins of the medical systems. All the *rtsa* of the medical system are said to originate from the main psychic veins.

According to Tibetan medicine these three columns are the first channels to originate in the embryo, and within eight weeks all the main chakras and the subtle psychic nerves have been formed.

Five other important veins which are the same in the medical as well as the tantric system are those which come off of the heart center or heart chakra. These are the veins of the various consciousnesses.

The first of these is the vein connected with the sense consciousness—of tasting, touching, hearing, smelling, and seeing; they are called the " five doors" and themselves branch off as five separate sense veins. The second is connected with the consciousness of one's ego sense; the third with mental consciousness—registering incoming impressions; the fourth with the store consciousness; and the fifth with transcendental consciousness.

The latter is the most important vein, the vein of realization. It runs through the heart and corresponds to the subtle central channel. In Tibetan psychiatry, it is said that if the other consciousnesses or the other pathways of the humors insert into the space of the transcendental consciousness vein, then insanity results. This will be taken up in more detail later in the psychiatry section.

In this system of subtle physiology, the tantric and medical systems meet in the theory and practice of healing. For example, the purification of the channels and the psychic airs by various breathing exercises affects the subtle body and physical levels of oxygen within the organism. When the subtle body is invigorated and strengthened, it imparts strength and lustre to the physical body. The breathing exercises affect the humoral airs in the physical body. The pathways are cleared so that the various airs can circulate harmoniously without obstruction. Further, such exercises give the tantric practitioner control of otherwise autonomous functions of the body—like regulation of heart beat and inner heat.

By keeping the channels straight, the psychic force or winds naturally flow in a proper way; when this happens, mind naturally relaxes into a state of ease or comfort. Thus, posture can affect the mind, and this is why one never sees a hunched-over yogi. It is especially important that the spine be kept straight when doing yogic breathing exercises.

Through the yogic control of breath the outer airs of the external world and inner airs of the subtle world are harmonized within the body. Healing takes place in this way, so also does the development of psychic powers.

The subtle and physical bodies are replicas and reflections of each other. Instead of having the solid form of matter, the subtle body has the radiant form of energy. Its brightness and density changes with our thoughts and feelings. Sickness can be seen by someone who is sensitive to its light and color as dark areas and grey smokey colors obscuring the natural radiance of health.

The Chakras and The Splendid Inner Vision

The chakras or psychic plexuses (Tib. *khor-lo,* literally "wheel") are the circular centers formed on the central column by the intersection of many subtle veins and the collection of various essences. When the chakras are purified and fully opened, they become the internal mandalas of the Five Innate Buddhas.

The number of veins at each psychic center accounts for the number of petals or spokes of the wheel associated with each chakra. The colors, sounds, elements, etc. associated with each chakra reflect the specific aspects of consciousness which the chakra represents. The chakras are progressively more refined starting from the lowest center, which represents sexual energy, up to the topmost chakra related to pure awareness. The lowest center flowers first and without much effort. Since there is so much pleasure at this center, it creates an inertial force which many people never care to move beyond. However, there are tantric practices that use the force of the sexual center to realize the non-dual bliss of wisdom.

In the Tibetan tantric system there is a maximum of six major chakras, as opposed to the seven in the Hindu system. Usually only

THE CHAKRAS

	Head Chakra	Throat Chakra	Heart Chakra	Navel Chakra	Genital Chakra
Tibetan name	Wheel of Bliss	Wheel of Enjoyment	Wheel of Phenomena	Wheel of Transmutation	Wheel of the Preservation of Happiness
Number of spokes	32	16	8	64	32
Bija	OM	AH	HUM	SWA	HA
Color	White	Red	Blue	Yellow	Green
Element	Ether/space	Fire	Water	Earth	Air
Direction	Center	West	East	South	North
Buddha Family	Buddha	Padma (lotus)	Vajra	Ratna (jewel)	Karma
Dhyani-Buddha	Vairocana, literally "Who Makes Forms Visible"	Amitabha, literally "Boundless Light"	Akshobhya, literally "Imperturable"	Ratnasambhava, literally, "Origin of Jewels"	Amoghasiddhi, literally, "Infallible Success"
Buddha Aspect	Body	Speech	Mind	Quality	Activity
Vehicle	Lion	Peacock	Elephant	Horse	Shang-shang bird
Skandha	Forms	Perceptions	Consciousness	Feelings	Concepts
Poison	Ignorance	Desire	Anger	Pride	Jealousy
Wisdom (transmuted poison)	Dharmadhatu Absolute Wisdom	Discriminating Wisdom	Mirror Wisdom	Equalizing Wisdom	All-accomplishing Wisdom
Gland	Pineal and pituitary	Thyroid	Adrenal	Pancreas (?)	Gonads

five chakras are used in Tibetan inner visualization, and often only three are mentioned. When only three are used, they always correspond to the centers of Buddha body, Buddha speech, and Buddha mind. They are referred to as "the three places."

The chakra of body is in the spot between the eyebrows. It is associated with white light and the transmutation of ignorance. The chakra of speech is at the throat and is associated with red light and the transmutation of desire. The chakra of mind is at the heart and is associated with blue light and the transmutation of anger.

The fourth chakra is the navel chakra of quality. It is a yellow light and represents the transmutation of ego. The fifth chakra is the genital center of activity. It is associated with green light, and represents the transmuation of jealousy.

In some practices, it is the whole top of the skull that is referred to as the head chakra, the "crown chakra," instead of the place between the eyes. When both head chakras are mentioned, it makes a total of six. The medical system includes all six.

The chart on page 74 sums up much of the basic information on the five chakras. As such, it reflects the precise correspondences which Buddhist tantra describes between ordinary mental, energetic, and physical functions and their counterparts in Buddha-nature.

By practice of tantric visualization and exercises leading eventually to realization, this transformation of one's own body into the mandalas of the Buddhas is the apotheosis of tantric practice. Its description is the inner vision and experience of the path to enlightenment through the human body.

In Tibetan religious literature, one often comes across stories of men and women who appear to be ordinary people but who are actually emanations (or the realization) of Buddhahood. When these people are cut open, as they somehow come to be in the stories, whole realms of glorious luminous deities and mandalas and whole networks and webs of glistening energy patterns are revealed within their bodies.

In general there are said to be forty-two peaceful deities residing in a mandala at the heart center and the fifty-eight wrathful deities in a mandala at the head center. In addition there are ten lineage deities, the gurus of the initiate's tradition, in the throat. The peaceful deities respond to our intuitive, feeling capacities. If we can't relate directly on that level, the enlightened energy has to bounce back on us in a wrathful way—which we can comprehend with our intellectual faculties. Such terrifying demeanor of the awesome deities cuts through our cold wall of intellectual protection and forces an emotive reaction which has the effect of reintegrating the intuitive and intellectual aspects of ourselves.

In terms of the medicine mandala, the highest or "secret" way of approaching it is to internalize it in this tantric way. The *Gyu-zhi* instructs us to visualize the center of the medicine mandala, the Medicine Buddha himself, residing in our head chakra. The medicine mountains of the four directions of the mandala are likewise at the other chakras. As previously described, these mountains represent a basic four-fold division of means of maintaining health and curing disease. The western Mt. Malaya which maintains the vital organs is at the throat chakra; the eastern Mt. Ponadan which cures every disease is at the heart chakra; the southern Mt. Begche which neutralizes heat is at the navel chakra; and the northern Mt. Gangchen which neutralizes cold is at the genital chakra.

Thus, the realization of the three bodies of Buddhahood in general or in specific aspects is the result of the tantric yoga of the subtle body.

Buddhist tantric yoga is divided into two stages: the accumulating (kye-rim) stage and the perfecting (dzog-rim) stage. These involve, respectively, rituals and yogic procedures. Beyond both of them is the highest yoga of the Vajrayana, Ati-yoga. It has no object of concentration, no objective references to be manipulated and transformed. It is the direct realization of the Buddha-nature, the immediate experience of enlightenment, the union of awareness (Tib. *rig-pa*) and emptiness (Tib. *stong-pa nyid*).

Tantric Ritual Healing and Medicines

Vajrayana techniques of realizing Buddha-nature by identifying oneself with a deity have specific applications and forms related to medicine. One group of these is the tantric rituals that a lama or practitioner performs in order to heal others. The second is the process of self-healing, curing oneself with tantric methods.

Spiritual or Dharmic medicines (Tib. *chos-sman*) are produced in tantric rituals in order to heal the sick. They are specifically the kinds of religious medicine that can cure disease which is karmic in cause and which therefore cannot be affected by ordinary herbal medicines. The psychiatric chapters of the *Gyu-zhi* specifically call for this kind of medicine because psychiatric diseases are often caused by spiritual causes that are beyond the reach of "rational" or somatic medicine.

The "spiritual medicine" created in the tantric ritual is an essential component of the whole Tibetan medical system.

This spiritual medicine is called ambrosia, dutsi (Tib. *bdud-rtsi*). It is also known as "accomplishment medicine" (*sman-drub*) or mendrup. It is generated by the lama or tantric adept through the activation of the subtle vital essence, thigle, as the bodhi-mind. It can be comunicated to the ones to be healed in various ways. All of those, however, are forms of the blessings or "radiant connection-waves" (Tib. *byin-gyis-rlabs*).

This medicine may be a pill or it may be drops of water which the lama sprinkles on the people or it may be communicated by the lama's touch, by hearing his sounds or even just by seeing him when he is in the transformed state, identified with the meditation deity (yidam).

There are many forms of tantric medicine, but the essence of its power is that the adept has completely transformed himself into the Buddha-deity and can therefore communicate the healing aspect of Buddha-power.

Any tantric deity can be invoked for healing purposes, a wrathful or peaceful deity depending on the exigency of the situation and the tantrika's own practice. For example, exorcism of an "evil spirit" causing a disease needs a wrathful deity, but the basic tantric formula for creating Dharma-medicine is the same.

The lama begins, after taking refuge and generating the bodhicitta for the sake of all beings, by visualizing a mantric seed-syllable emerging from the open space of voidness. This seed syllable represents the manifest essence of the meditational deity.

The meditational deity is projected in the space before one or on top of one's head (although sometimes it may immediately be visualized as oneself). The lights from the three places of the deity— head, throat and heart centers—are absorbed by one's own three centers. The lights streaming in at the forehead center purify the body, karmic actions and the subtle channels; at the throat center they purify speech, emotional defilements and the *rlung;* at the heart center they purify mind, mental obscurations and the thigle essences. At the fourth center, the navel center or again at the heart, they purify the inborn habits and subtle tendencies, awakening the absolute Buddha qualities.

By virtue of the purification of the chakras, the poisons associated with each chakra are drawn out. The airs held in at the base of the central column where the three main veins meet activates the red-drop bodhi essence (Tib. *bdud-rtsi byang-sems dmar-po*) there, and it generates heat that burns away the poisons. The purified energies of the chakras are turned into deities in mandalas. The heat from the mother thigle reaches the crown chakra where the white condensed radiant pearl-drop bodhi-essence (*bdud-rtsi byang-sems dkar-po*) melts or descends from the head down the central column and pervades the whole being of the practitioner. It is at this point that the lama is fully empowered to create the healing blessings.

Whatever form the Dharma medicine takes, the person who takes it shares in the radiant communication-waves of blessing and is therefore bound by a vow or pledge (Tib. *dam-tshig*). The vow is the actual precepts of the ritual but, existentially, it is the bond created in the open space of awareness between the lama-deity and the person healed. Breaking this sort of bond is considered a major cause of disease by Tibetans. The meaning of the *dam-tshig* actually goes beyond the formal ritual bond. It means all the promises and spiritual truths we have recognized in moments of heightened awareness, peak moments, as it were, and especially those in relation to the lama. To go against these and to cause any obstacles between oneself and the lama is to be highly self-destructive on the most meaningful level and therefore disease ensues.

In this kind of healing tantric ritual, which William Stablein has so well described in his work,[49] there are usually three kinds of medicine created, and these correspond to the outer, inner, and secret levels of disease. The outer one is a pill made of eight Ayurvedic ingredients charged with the blessing of the deity. The inner one is torma (*gtor-ma*), ritual offering cake. These torma are made in the shapes of ears, nose, etc. and they represent the body purified by the eight inner substances which promote bodily growth. The secret medicine is represented by eight sexual aspects of the subtle body, four from the male and four from the female.

Sometimes the Dharma medicines made by great lamas are taken before death, during the process of dying, in order to affect the spiritual health of the consciousness at that most critical time—when the quality of consciousness so dramatically affects the journey through the stages before rebirth and the level of the rebirth itself.

In terms of visualizing the medicine mandala for the healing of others, it is approached in the intermediate or "inner" way. This means one should visualize oneself as the Medicine Buddha and the outer world as the medicine mandala. This is the practice of purifying perception of the world and the self, transforming both into their

Buddha-nature. In this case, one is always generating the healing rays of the Medicine Buddha, always generating the best of one's emotional and intellectual capacity as compassion and wisdom in their healing aspects. Realizing the whole of the outer world in its Buddha-nature, it all becomes medicine.

The Vajrayana or Tantrayana path is also called the Mantrayana, the way of using primordial mystic syllables called mantras as a means of salvation. Thus there is a tantric way of healing with mantras.

The subtle body is the energy body and energy is manifested as vibration. In the impure, unrealized, and diseased body, the vibrational sounds are discordant and unclear.

Eliade has called the tantric ritual or sadhana "a gnostic system and an internalized liturgy."[50] The inner litany is the sound of mantras, the vibrational expression of manifest Buddha-nature.

By practicing the recitation of mantras, one can readjust the vibrational harmony of the subtle body and realize it as the Buddha-body. But learning a mantra out of a book and practicing it without empowerment doesn't usually work. Most mantras must be received in initiation from the master or lama either in actual experience or by more mystical means. Further, mantras have no power if they are repeated mindlessly like a parrot.

Depending on the ailment, different mantras are prescribed to help one "tune in" to the inherent Buddha-nature. There is a mantra of the Medicine Buddha which can be used in all cases. Mantras are thus particularly used in the healing of mental disorders since they can readjust the vibrations of consciousness.

Special forms of mantric healing rely on the occult correspondence between the mystic syllables and the subtle veins of the body. In one healing process of the Vajrayana tradition, certain mantric syllables are said to mark the points where the intricate systems of subtle veins criss-cross each other. When the syllables are not clear, disease results. At these points on the veins the vibration has become blocked, and the flesh at those points may become hardened as a result. The mantric sounds are said to exist within the psychic veins blended with the airs (and mind, as we have noted, rides the winds). Meditation on these mantras at the crossed points or knots of the veins clears the syllable and cures the disease. This is a very advanced and subtle form of healing. As applied to self-healing, it can only be done by someone who has very strong powers of meditation.[51]

Other examples of mantric healing practices are visualizing a special healing mantra in the form of a mandala on one's own hand so that the hand has special healing powers of touch and visualizing the healing mantric mandala in the heart of the person to be cured.

Besides the manifestation of life and consciousness as the sounds of mantra within the subtle body, the other primary manifestation is of light. The visualization of light is central to tantric sadhanas and to tantric healing. One visualizes the deity radiating rays of light that

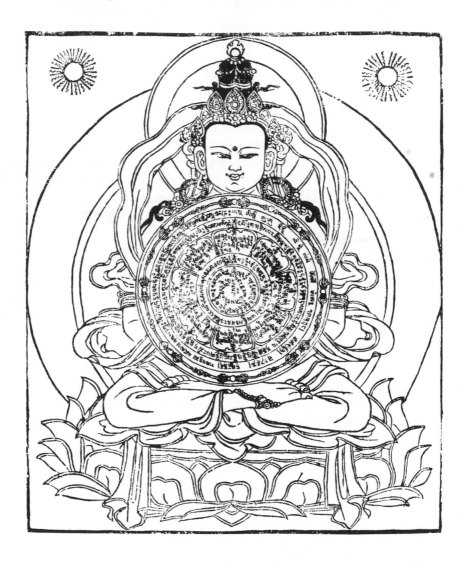

Figure 13 Amitayus, Tsepame, the Buddha of Immortal Life. Visualization of this deity and recitation of his mantra are spiritual medicine believed to gather the blessings that prolong life and prevent disease and untimely death. The mandala he holds is made of the syllables of his long-life mantra.

enter oneself and others, completely purifying mental and physical obscurations and disease. Then the deity merges into oneself at one's heart center in the form of light. This light destroys dualistic conception, and one dwells in the state of radiant emptiness. Upon emerging from the meditation on the void, one is fully identified with the deity and can again send rays of healing light to the sick person. One can also concentrate on healing oneself with the visualization of the light.

All this points to the fact that Tibetan medicine strongly emphasizes the state of mind of the healer as a major part of the healing process. In the Tibetan view, the healer's state of mind is not just a moral question which has no effect on the patient. It is held to be a vitally important influence on his condition. The ability to effect spiritual cures depends on the healer's consciousness—his meditative powers of concentration and his purity of intention. Therefore, whatever kind of medicine is being practiced, the Tibetan healer will also be practicing internally various mystic healing exercises, visualizations, mantras, etc.

Jewels also are used in healing to adjust the inner light of the subtle body. Gem therapy was known in Vedic times when jewels were used in ash form as medicines. Gems are believed to be mines of radiations containing the power of one of seven aspects of light, the cosmic energy as manifested from the diamond-like void into rainbow light. The seven-fold spectrum of light in the rainbow represents the basic energies, forces, and quality of the manifest world. Therefore gems operate on the same kind of subtle level as the subtle body which is, of course, referred to on its realized level as the rainbow body.

At the center of the medicine mandala in the crystal palace of the Medicine Buddha there are three kinds of gems: gods' gems, bodhisattvas' gems, humans' gems. The first are said to have the power to give rebirth in heavenly realms; the second, the power to "lift up dead men to nirvana" and to help people to understand Dharma; and the third, the power to counteract poisons, evil spirits, swellings, and fevers.

Jewels connect the purely spiritual medicine mandala with the substantial reality of manifestation and disease. In the *Gyu-zhi* gems are said to solve all the problems of the three humors that cause the 404 diseases and to afford protection from the 1,080 evil spirits. In terms of religion, the "Three Jewels," the Buddha, Dharma, and Sangha, are said to fulfill all desires of sentient beings and thus to be the "wish-fulfilling gem."

Tibetan healers wear gems for protection against negative forces, especially those radiating from the patient. This category of subtle medicines and preventative measures also include many kinds of amulets which are usually made by lamas and which are imparted with the tantric blessings. These include protection cords and little packages of specially empowered mantras and blessed objects. Sometimes even the medicine pills themselves are worn in the little sealed case around the neck. Relics from Lord Buddha himself and from other high realized beings are also in this category. One especially precious relic is a little pearl-like substance that is found among the ashes of great lamas after they have been cremated.

There are also physical methods of treatment that affect the subtle body. One such method is acupuncture. Another is massage. Through massage the healer is charging the subtle body with the life force he has gained control of in himself. He combines this with visualizations. He is also more sensitive to various energy blockages in the other person because he has controlled his own mind and can therefore tune into the other person mentally, subtly and physically. Circular strokes are said to charge the area with energy and lengthwise strokes are said to discharge poisons and blockages.

A special kind of message called "kunyi" (Tib. *bsku-mnye*), literally "ointment massage," is used to relax tensions within the subtle body and to break up the "knots" where energies have become solidified due to blockage in the channels.

Aromatic medicinal substances in oils or butter are applied in conjunction with massage. The Tibetans maintain that consciousness can be affected through the skin where the path of the airs (and thus of the mind) interfaces with the external environment.

Finally, breathing exercises serve to strengthen the life wind and clear the channels in the subtle body and thus generate good health to the physical body from within. Through special breathing practice and visualizations the outer airs are used to activate the subtle inner elements, and this brings about psychic powers, including the power of healing.

Self-Healing and The Meditation of the Medicine Buddha

Any person who is practicing Vajrayana Buddhism but who does not have full or even highly developed meditative powers and realization may still use some tantric techniques for healing himself. Ultimately self-healing is aimed at the religious definition of complete health: full enlightenment. On a more relative plane, however, a person can deal with his illness by using Dharma practice for self-healing.

It is of primary importance that anyone who wishes to do self-healing must fully understand that one's disease is symptomatic of a fundamental spiritual disharmony in some aspect of one's own life in and of itself or in relationship to other beings and the environment. Therefore, one has to cultivate a healing attitude from within.

The main attitude that has to be generated is that illness is a blessing. It is first of all a signal that something we are doing is fundamentally off balance. Having gotten the signal, we can readjust the balance to create harmony. There is no guilt or self-blame implied in this—such feelings would simply be more obstructions generated by delusion and become a further cause of anxiety and disease. But it is necessary to be completely honest and open with ourselves. The sickness, then, provides an opportunity to grow, to see where we've gone wrong (out of balance), to recognize our past negative acts, and to practice self-development through self-healing.

In other words, our illness provides us with an opportunity to practice taking suffering as the path of Dharma, to practice using suffering as a support for Dharma in specific ways, like thinking that by this difficulty one is gaining greater opportunity to progress in Dharma, to intensify the aspiration toward enlightenment, to transmute the suffering in awareness. It is also a support for developing compassion, practicing virtue, overcoming pride, purifying defilements and for releasing oneself from the aversion to pain and unhappiness.

As the third Dodrup Chen Rinpoche wrote on the subject:

> Whenever harm comes to you from beings or non-beings, if your mind experiences only the consciousness of sorrow, then even from a small incident great mental pain will develop. For it is its nature that any consciousness, either of suffering or happiness, will increase by experiencing it. If the experience gradually becomes stronger, a time will come when most of what appears will become the cause of drawing unhappiness to ourselves, and happiness will never have a chance. If you do not know that the responsibility lies with one's own mind's way of experiencing, and you

put the blame on external objects alone, then the ceaseless flame of suffering and anger-bad karma will increase. That is called 'appearances arising in the form of an enemy.'

Therefore, not to be hurt by the obstacles of enemies, illness, and harmful spirits does not mean that we can drive away vicissitudes such as illness, and that they won't occur again. Rather it means that they will not be able to arise and take the form of obstacles to the practice of the Path of Enlightenment.[52]

Tantric rituals are used to give a person who is doing self-healing an outer structure on which to project inner strength. The strength is identified with the deity. It purifies oneself, is reabsorbed, enlarged and fully identified with—oneself becomes the deity. The aspects of the subtle body thus identified with the cosmic powers of Buddhahood are put to work healing the illness. The main part of such practice is to visualize brilliant light streaming from the deity and directing it to the particular place to be cured, if that is necessary, or simply, in general, streaming throughout the body, purifying and transforming it. White light and blue light are most often used for healing purposes. In the healing of others the circulated light does not just remain in oneself but is radiated out into the ordinary universe— purifying and healing all beings.

The act of recognizing our mental defilements and transgressions and the way of purifying them is usually accomplished through ritual meditation on the Buddha Vajrasattva. Vajrasattva (Dorje Sempa) is the special deity whose aspect of Buddha-nature is that purification. The practice is to visualize him on top of the head. He is pure white in color, sitting in lotus posture, holding in his left hand by his hip a bell symbolizing wisdom and in his right hand by his heart a vajra symbolizing skillful means. He is smiling gently and is sublimely beautiful. One confesses one's "sins" before him, and such a ritual confession has great psychological benefit.

Then by the power of our faith and the resolve not to commit the transgressions again, and through the strength of our meditation as well as his vow to save and purify, the light from the mantra spinning in his heart, which is radiating out to the Buddhas of the universe and returning their light to him, drops into us through the top of the head and our internal body becomes luminous. We visualize all our negative emotions, physical sickness, and mental obscurations, all our bad karma and habitual dispositions, as passing out of us in the forms of blood and pus, dark smoke, horrible insects and spiders, all of which satisfy the lords of karmic debt who wait hungrily below.

While meditation on Vajrasattva can be used for self-healing, there are many other deities who may also be invoked for curing disease, and supreme among them is the Medicine Buddha, Sangye Menla, the Radiant Lord of Healing.

Anyone who wishes to do so can practice the meditation of the Medicine Buddha. The general method of doing the practice will be described here according to the instructions of Dudjom Rinpoche. It can be used for healing oneself and others.[53]

One must begin any practice with the sections of refuge and bodhicitta; that is, taking refuge in the Three Jewels and developing the inspiration and action to produce the thought of enlightenment for both oneself and others.

From the state of voidness before the mind is interrupted by other thoughts, visualize the syllable AH emerging in the space before you. AH represents the state that is free from birth, exhaustion and concept; its nature is shunyata. The syllable AH becomes the form of the Medicine Buddha, the object of concentration.

The Medicine Buddha is radiant, translucent, blue in color, holding the myrobalan plant in the fingers of his right hand, which is extended on his knee in the gesture of giving. His left hand rests in his lap and holds a begging bowl filled with healing nectar. He is dressed in the three monastic robes and sits in the full lotus posture on a thousand-petalled lotus which itself sits on a jeweled throne.

Imagine the place where you are meditating as a Buddha-field with a beautiful landscape. The whole of space is filled with rainbow lights and offering deities and goddesses who hold objects of offering—everything that is beautiful and pleasing to the senses. Mentally make all the most precious offerings you can imagine to the Medicine Buddha. Invite him to bestow his blessings and to sit on the top of your head. Pray that he bestow his healing power. There are many different prayers that might be said, but basically recitation of his mantra is the most essential. The mantra of the Medicine Buddha is: TEYATA: OM BEKANZE BEKANZE MAHABEKANZE BE-KANZE RAZA SAMUDGATE SWAHA.[54] Repeat the mantra as much as you can.

Recite the mantra with one-pointed concentration and devotion and with the intention that healing occur. From the heart center of the Medicine Buddha where the mantra is spinning clockwise, rays of light as bright as one hundred rising suns radiate out into yourself and

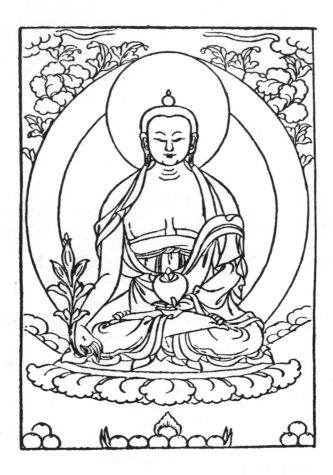

Figure 14 A woodcut of the Medicine Buddha from a contemporary medical handbook. The meditation practice of the Medicine Buddha is used to relieve all kinds of mental and physical suffering. The teaching, which Manjushri received from the Buddha, eventually came to Abbot Shantarakshita, who established a lineage of its practice in Tibet beginning in the eighth century; from then until recent years it was practiced continuously at Samye Monastery. The saintly pandita Atisha brought a different tradition of it to Tibet in the 11th century, and there are other lineages as well. Therefore there are different visualizations and longer or short versions of the mantra, but the essence of the practice is the same.

others, dispelling disease and suffering and even the cause of suffering. The lights touch all beings and their darkness disappears, likewise all their suffering. Visualize in this way while reciting the mantra.

Afterwards, visualize yourself and all beings dissolving into a state of emptiness. Try to remain in that space totally free from thoughts and any concept of subject, object and action. This is the absolute way of practice. This is mingling with the state of the Medicine Buddha's mind.

Re-emerging from this state, see all thoughts as sharing the nature of the Medicine Buddha's mind, perceive all sounds as his mantra and all forms as his manifestation. Then mentally dedicate the merit and good karma accrued from this practice to the enlightenment of all beings.

The most important aspect of this meditation, the essence of the healing practice, is to have strong selfless compassion for others and to have fervent trust and complete confidence in the sadhana practice, in the deity. Without confidence in the Medicine Buddha, the practice of his meditation will not help.

If you are concerned with the healing of specific people or animals, mentally visualize them receiving the light of the Medicine Buddha and repeat the mantra with them in mind. Send the light to any specific part of the body that needs healing. If you are taking or giving actual medications and medicines, consider them as the nectar of the Medicine Buddha. If you are practicing medicine of any form, whether surgery or massage, always consider that the Medicine Buddha is sitting on top of your head and radiating great healing light to the patient. Always recite the mantra, either out loud or silently. Combining this mental and spiritual practice of the Medicine Buddha with other forms of medicine will greatly enhance the force of healing.

Summary

In summing up the Tibetan tantric healing, we can say that it involves visualization of the subtle body and control of subtle energy forces and essences. Through purification and manipulation, the vital essence and the life forces inherent in the airs flowing through the psychic channels and chakras are transformed into bodhi-mind and wisdom-truth.

Tantric rituals and yogic techniques (visualizations, breathing exercises, mantras, etc.) are the means by which control of the so-called subtle body is gained. The subtle body is an invisible energy form that shapes and generates the physical body.

In order to do tantric healing one must have developed concentration and awareness through the practice of meditation and Dharma. The psychic powers gained in tantric practice are never acquired for their own sake. They are the instruments of compassion and emptiness, wisdom and skillful means. This is of the utmost importance. Without the crucial right intention—for the sake of easing the suffering of all beings and bringing them the happiness (health) of Buddhahood—then the psychic powers of tantra are dangerous, evil, selfish, in short, everything producing sickness and suffering. Intention is the most important basis in the practice of Dharma and in the practice of Tibetan medicine in all its three main aspects. Right intention is the bodhicitta. It is said that whatever we do, if we do it with the right intention, then we are practicing Dharma and helping other beings.

By the methods of tantra the seemingly "miraculous" cures of psychic and spiritual healing take place. In actuality they are not miraculous but are supernatural in the sense that they involve the subtle penetration of the universal forces of life and consciousness concentrated within the microcosm of the body.

Through tantric techniques lama-healers make powerful Dharma medicines, medicines which transfer the cosmic energy-purity of the Buddhas to the sick. Some of these medicines have no substantial forms, but are rather sounds, smells, appearances. All create a bond, the samaya, between healer, patient, and deity.

Tantric self-healing is a way of applying the healing practices of tantra to oneself. In its advanced forms its effectiveness depends on the meditative powers of the individual. In a more basic way, however, it can be done by anyone on the path. Its essence is turning suffering and sickness into the opportunity to advance spirituality. Visualizations for purification and healing are included here. To do self-healing is not, however, to abandon medicine. The idea is to combine spiritual healing with regular medicine to get the full effect.

6

Somatic Medicine: Basic Descriptive Aspects

According to Tibetan medicine, the essence of health is holistic harmony. It is a harmony of formless, subtle and manifest worlds, of mental, emotional and physical bodies, of spiritual, psychological and organic developments, of self, others and total environment.

In the view of Tibetan medicine the microcosm of the body and the macrocosm of the universe are constantly dancing with each other. When they are out of step with each other or when they are out of tune with the spiritual reality that sets them moving, disease results.

The five elements are what unite the macrocosm and the microcosm. All things, animate and inanimate, share the same material basis—the five great elements: earth, water, fire, wind, and space. These are cosmic principles, cosmic energies, sometimes even described as sub-atomic cosmo-physical theory, rather than being just the simple things their names imply. For example, water is said to contain all five elements.

Since these five are all-pervading principles of phenomena, they are called "great": earth is the principle of solidifying or forming, water the principle of cohesion, fire of ripening or maturing, and wind of preserving (for example, a body without *rlung* decays); space supports these four.

In the body, the gross physical elements are expressed as follows: flesh and bones are earth, blood and lymph are water, body heat is fire, nervous and motor function is wind, and consciousness is space. As extremely subtle inner elements, they are described in terms of very refined energies expressed as five-colored lights. These subtle inner elements arise from the primordially luminous void wisdom mind; the gross physical elements arise from the subtle inner elements.

The entire Buddhist medical system is based on the reciprocal principle of the five elements. The art of healing involves maintaining homeostasis within the internal functions of the body and between the outer environment. A specific disease and the medicine prescribed for it will have the same basic material composition of elements. The three humors of the body also share the underlying nature of the five elements.

In order to comprehend the Tibetan tradition of medical psychiatry it is necessary to be acquainted with the fundamental principles and terms of the system of general medicine, for medical psychiatry is grounded in it. What follows is an outline of the basic theory of disease, diagnosis, and treatment which will be elaborated on later as they relate to psychiatry.

The Humoral Theory

The principal idea of health that emerges in Tibetan medicine is that of balance, balance within the body and between it and its corresponding aspects in the outer world. In terms of the body, that balance is primarily expressed as the harmony of the three humors— wind, bile and phlegm.

The three humors (Tib. *nyes-pa;* Skt. *dosha,* literally "fault") originate on a spiritual plane from the basic mental confusion that produces subject-object dualism and thus the karmic force to manifest life and the universe. Ignorance, desire, and aversion evolve into the humors phlegm, air, and bile respectively. Once produced, the balanced circulation of these humors on their own course maintains the health of the organism. The three humors are the principle triad in Tibetan somatic medicine.

The humoral theory is taken directly from Indian Ayurvedic medicine and Indian Buddhist philosophy. "Humor" is an insufficient translation but the standard one, it being an archaic term for "moisture" that was applied to Greco-Roman humoral medicine. However, humor means "subtle principle" of life energies as well as actual bodily constituents or fluids.

It is also rather difficult to translate the words for each of the three humors. Wind, bile, and phlegm are the standard translations, but these hardly indicate that they are pervasive principles, neither do they parallel a modern view of the body or biochemistry. For example, the term *rlung* translated as "wind" or "air" does not just mean the gases of the stomach or intestines or the function of breath, although it includes them. It may help to realize that *rlung* can also be thought of as "force" or "pressure," and also that *rlung* has a direct relationship with mind or psychological states. A stress disorder such as high blood pressure is considered a *rlung* disease.

The humor *rlung* controls such diverse functions as breathing, spitting, muscular activity, speech, menstruation, urination and relaying sensory input. It is the humor directly related to mind and is always involved in mental or emotional illness. Since this *rlung*—air, wind, pressure, energy, force—is said to control the other two humors and can also mix with them (it is neutral while they are not), this indicates that in Tibetan medicine there is always a psychosomatic aspect or possibility in any disease.

mKhris-pa, which is translated as "bile," does not mean just the secretion of the liver, although it includes that—and liver disorders like jaundice are considered bile diseases. "Bile" seems to indicate the whole of digestive metabolism, vital energy, and heat.

Finally, *bad-kan,* which is translated as "phlegm," while including the maintenance and accumulation of mucus throughout the body—and asthma is a disease of phlegm—does not mean only that. It may also relate to the lymphatic system and infectious diseases in general—tuberculosis, for example, is a phlegm disease. It will remain to Western doctors who study Tibetan medicine to decide exactly how the humors correspond to modern medical theory.

A contemporary Tibetan doctor has explained a modern view of the three humors as follows:[55]

The humor air is the vital force. It is understood to be concentrated in the nucleus; it controls metabolism.

The humor bile is the vital energy. It is understood as the energy released during catabolic activity by enzymatic reactions.

The humor phlegm is understood as the anabolic force which synthesizes new protoplasm.

The vital force (air) controls both catabolism and anabolism. It resides in the nucleus of each cell. Diseases depend first on imbalance in this vital force. Diseases of anabolic force (phlegm) and vital energy (bile) are mixed with the vital force.

The vital force, air, has five divisions which circulate through the body. The vital energy (bile) is divided into two kinds: fine and bigger. The fine vital energy resides in the cells; the larger resides in the whole body and also has five divisions. The anabolic force, phlegm, has five divisions as well, and is spread throughout the body.

In the classical terms of Tibetan medicine, each humor has five divisions and seats, as well as certain qualities, times, places, psychological and physiological types associated with it. Specific details of the three humors are put together in the following charts (more information is also found in the outline of the "Tree of Health and Disease" later in this chapter).

	WIND/AIR (Tib. *rlung;* "lung"; Skt. *vayu*)
Subtle Principle:	Mind
Quality:	Dry, light, cold, subtle, volatile, pungent, soft.
Production encouraged by:	Desire, attachment and lust; spiritual development in both positive and negative aspects, aceticism, sexual repression, lack of sleep and food, deliberate withholding of natural eliminative processes.
Five Types:	1. *Srog-'dzin*—"life accompanying wind" — assists breathing—seat in heart center.[56]
	2. *Gyen-rgyu*—"upward moving wind" — assists speech—seat in chest, but travels to nose and gullet.
	3. *Khyab-byed*—"pervasive wind" — assists muscular motion — seat in head but travels to all parts of body.
	4. *Me-mnyam*—"fire-accompanying wind" — assists digestion and assimilation—seat in abdomen but travels to all parts of intestines and stomach.
	5. *Thur-sel*—"downward clearing wind" — assists excretion — seat in "secret" genital center but travels to intestines, bladder, sexual organs, and thighs.
Body and character type:	Crooked bodies, thin and bluish in complexion. Joints produce cracking sounds. Susceptible to cold breezes. Fond of singing, laughing, talking, arguing, fighting. Fond of bitter and sour and hot food. Shortest life span of the three types.
Main Seat:	Lower part of body, abdomen.

Season:	Air diseases accumulated in spring, break out in summer, subside in autumn.
Effect of intoxicating drugs:	Craziness.
Geographical:	Cold and windy places like Russia and Tibet encourage the production of air and give rise to air disturbances.
Time:	Rising periods of air are evening and pre-dawn.
Symbolized by:	Vulture.

BILE (Tib. *mkhris-pa,* "tripa"; Skt. *pitta*)

Subtle Principle:	Energy
Quality:	Hot, oily, light, violent, slightly unctuous, musty, liquid, flowing.
Production encouraged by:	Anger, hatred and aversion; changes of climate and excessive heat.
Five Types:	1. *'Ju-byed*—"digestive" — seat below stomach and above intestines. 2. *mDangs-sgyur*—"color transforming" — seat in liver. 3. *sGrub-byed*—"accomplishing" — seat in heart. 4. *mThong-byed*—"visually adjusting" — seat in eyes. 5. *mDog-gsal*—"complexion clearing" — seat in skin.
Body and character type:	Eats little but feels full, then feels hunger and thirst at frequent intervals. Yellow skin tone. Medium size and height. Proud and intelligent. Clear minded. Likes sweet and bitter food.
Main Seat:	Region between heart and adomen, center of body. When disturbed and imbalanced, it travels up and gives rise to fever. Air aggravates and worsens bile disease, then it travels all over body.
Season:	Bile diseases accumulate in summer, break out in autumn, subside in winter.
Effect of intoxicating drugs:	Extreme rough and coarse behavior.
Geographical:	Hot and dry countries (like the Arab countries and the plains of India) encourage production of bile.
Time:	Rising periods of bile are mid-day and mid-night.
Symbolized by:	Horse and mule.

PHLEGM (Tib. *bad-kan*, "bekan"; Skt. *kapha*)	
Subtle Principle:	Matter.
Quality:	Cold, heavy, sticky, sluggish, soft, slimy, and solid.
Production encouraged by:	Spiritual ignorance and physical sloth; over-indulgence in sleep and comfort; damp environment.
Five Types:	1. *rTen-byed*—"supportive"—seat in chest. 2. *Myag-byed*—"mixing"—seat in upper digestive tract. 3. *Myong-byed*—"experiencing" — seat in tongue. 4. *Tshim-byed*—"satisfying" — seat in head. 5. *'Byor-byed*—"connecting" — seat in all body joints.
Body and character type:	Fat and pale. Body does not have required warmth. Lives long, becomes rich. Jolly, helpful and fond of sour food. Eats a lot but doesn't get hungry. Even when harmed, won't respond; much later, however, will answer back.
Main Seat:	Upper part of body.
Season:	Phlegm diseases accumulate in winter, break out in spring and subside in summer.
Effect of intoxicating drugs:	Here, lightens so has good effect.
Geographical:	Damp countries like Europe and America encourage phlegm production.
Time:	Rising periods of phlegm are twilight and morning.
Symbolized by:	Elephant and lion.

The practice of humoral medicine consists of knowing how to reconstitute the humoral balance by adding or subtracting qualifications of the humor through food, environment, herbal medicines and other treatments. Tibetan medicine specifies numerous qualities, tastes, and powers that are associated with the humors and with the animal, vegetable and mineral substances used as medicines.

Similarly, behavior and emotional states affect the humors. For example, anger increases bile and desire increases wind. Astrology and the cycles of time also figure importantly in Tibetan medicine; each humor is also associated with a particular daily period, yearly season and stage of life during which time it predominates. Bodily types and dispositions are also associated with the three humors. For example, babies have a great predominance of phlegm. This is reflected in their inactiveness, accumulation of mucus, and closed-mindedness—all attributes of phlegm. In the case of a baby, that is a normal predominance for that life stage, but in an adult, it would be a sickness due to an overabundance of phlegm. Among the prescriptions for such a condition would be massage and exercise to counter the inactivity, all the foods which limit phlegm and a course of medicines to do the same.

The humoral theory may sound simplistic, but actually it is very complex and subtle. Rarely does a disturbance involve simply one humor. It is usually a combination of humoral forces, further conditioned by whether the disease is of a hot or cold nature, or whether it is a primary or secondary imbalance of the humor, or whether psychological or perhaps environmental factors are involved. It is said to take at least seven years to grasp the deep meaning of the three humors.

In addition to balancing the humors themselves, there are other aspects of the body that must be balanced along with them to maintain health. The *Gyu-zhi* says that it is the balance or imbalance of three classifications of 1) humors, 2) constituents, and 3) excretions that causes the body to thrive or be overcome.

The primary excretions or impurities are three in number; they are urine, feces and perspiration. The constituents, also called the "supports" of life, are seven in number and are as follows:

1. Food. Saliva separates the food into nutritious constituents which are absorbed; the wastes are excreted as stool and urine.

2. Blood. Nutrition produces energy which goes to the liver and produces blood. Blood is said to wet the body and "hold the life." It is excreted in gall bile.

3. Flesh. Blood turns into flesh. It is discharged from the "nine holes" (nostrils, ears, anus, etc.).

4. Fat. Flesh nutrition turns into fat. Excretion is the earwax and greasiness of the body discharged as perspiration.

5. Bone. Nutrition from fat turns into bone. It is excreted as teeth, nails, and hair.

6. Marrow. The essence of bone turns into marrow. Its excretion is "sleep in eyes," stool, and dandruff.

7. "Semen." The essence of marrow turns into "semen." The essence of "semen" goes to the heart. Its excretion, "the seed of heritage," goes into the seminal fluid. "Semen" is the most highly

refined feature in the body. The brightness and radiance of the face is said to come from the essence of "semen" at the heart. From the years one to twelve the essence of "semen" supports the growth of the body. From twelve to fifty it goes to strength, or during pregnancy, to the breasts for milk. From fifty to one-hundred it goes to maintenance of the body.

"Semen" also plays an important role in tantric medicine where, on a subtle plane, the regenerative fluid is called *thig-le* and is the potential bodhi-essence. In both tantric and somatic medicine it has the quality of generating splendor from the heart. By "semen" Tibetans do not just mean the male seminal fluid which is the excretion called "seed of heritage," or the female "menstrual bood," by which they imply the ovum, but the vital essence-drops that are spread throughout the body in numerous subtle channels as the supports of life and consciousness. They may relate to endrocrine secretions, the intra-cellular genetic principle, and even neurojuices that are the biochemical correlates of mental function.

In addition to the components of the body as the three humors, seven constituents, and three excretions, there are listed five sense organs (of sight, hearing, taste, touch, and smell), six hollow organs (the stomach, large intestine, small intestine, gall bladder, urinary bladder, and seminal vesicle or uterus), and the five solid organs (heart, liver, lungs, spleen, and kidneys).

The brain, which is not mentioned in early Indian Ayurvedic classics, is mentioned in the *Gyu-zhi* as the seat of phlegm, "ignorance" and "mental dullness." This may relate to the spiritual view that the discursive thought process interferes with higher awareness—perhaps like the modern view of the brain as a filtering system which processes, inhibits and selects the information it allows into consciousness. In the Tibetan medical system the brain is usually added as the sixth organ of sense, thinking being a sense activity; the control of consciousness, on the other hand, is related to the heart center.

Causes of Disease

The causes of disease reflect the fact that the balance of the humors (along with the supports and excrements) has to be maintained not only within the body but also in accord with the forces of the natural environment and the psychological life of the individual.

There are two kinds of causes of disease: one, the long term cause—spiritual factors, the karma from past lives; and two, the short terms cause—factors in this present life. Among the short term causes of disease, there are four main categories: (1) seasonal changes; (2) evil spirits; (3) poison; and (4) habit and behavior.

The classic way of listing all the kinds of diseases is as follows:

1. karmic diseases (*gzhan-dbang sngon-nad*)
2. evil spirit diseases (*kun-brtags gdon-nad*)
3. current or immediate diseases (*ltar-snang 'phral-nad*)
4. life diseases (*yongs-grub tshe-nad*)

1. Karmic diseases. In the widest sense all diseases are caused by karma since the body itself is generated by the force of the three main obscurations. However, karmic diseases as specific illness are those which cannot be cured by regular medicines. Their cause is purely spiritual, bad karma from this or past lives, and the medicine must be spiritual. In such cases it is necessary for a person to do religious practice—mantras and prostrations for example, or to have a lama do rituals and meditations for him. Only a lama or a highly developed being can perceive the spiritual causes of disease but if a disease cannot be cured by means of regular medicines, then one can adjudge it to be a karmic disease.

2. Diseases of "evil spirits." Diseases caused by "evil spirits" are generally treated with religious medicines and rituals, especially exorcisms, in combination with herbal medicines and other treatments such as medicine-oil, massage and mantra pills. "Evil spirits" are one of the main causes of insanity and psychiatric disturbances.

3. Immediate diseases. These come and go quickly. In modern medical terminology they would be called "self-terminating illnesses." They don't necessarily need medical treatment since they will go away by themselves.

4. Life diseases. Life diseases are the main category that is treated by standard somatic Tibetan medicine. These demand treatment; if they are left untreated, the patient will get worse and may die. These are humoral imbalances caused by the ill effects of bad food, irregular and destructive behavior (lack of sleep, unvirtuous living, poisons intake, etc.), environmental factors and psychological factors.

For example, regarding psychological stress as a cause of physiological ailments in the class of life disorders, jealousy or pride, it is said, may result in high blood pressure. Loss of a loved one may result in arthritis, but food factors—like eating too much pork—may also cause arthritis. Relaxing after over-eating or going without shoes in winter increases phlegm; falling from a horse or sitting in the midday summer sun contribute to the cause of bile disorders; and forceful activity (verbal or physical) on an empty stomach can give rise to wind disorders.

These medically "treatable" diseases are first approached by naturopathy, by relying on the therapeutics of diet and behavior without any more elaborate treatment. This indicates the practical, basically common sense approach of the Tibetan medical system. A Tibetan doctor will always avoid extreme therapeutic measures whenever possible because of the potential ill effects these could have on other spheres of the individual's life, thereby imbalancing him further and possibly even more profoundly.

Fundamentally, Tibetan naturopathy is understood in terms of "tastes" and "powers" of foods and medicines that affect the seventeen qualifications associated with the three humors. There are six tastes: sweet, sour, salty, bitter, acrid and astringent; and three post-digestive tastes: sweet, sour and astringent. There are eight powers: heavy, greasy, cool, bland, light, coarse, hot and acute. Additionally, there are seventeen secondary qualities.

Great consideration is therefore given to diet since food has the ability to directly affect the humors. Understanding one's humoral disposition, the proper diet is prescribed as preventative medicine. In general, disorders of the digestive process are thought to be very serious and to precipitate disease. Regarding the amount of food to be eaten at each meal in order to maintain good health and mental clarity, Tibetan medicine follows the teaching of the Buddha on this point: the stomach should be one-third full with food, one-third full with liquids, and one-third empty.

Certain combinations of food are thought to be rather poisonous because each food strongly influences different humors, either negating the good qualities of each food or having a combined effect that is deleterious. For example, honey and peanuts together are not good because they negate each other—the power of honey to affect phlegm and of peanut butter to affect wind is diminished. The combinations of fish and milk, eggs and fish, or chicken and curd are said to be poisonous.

Behavior like sleeping in the day, irregular patterns of eating and sleeping, suppressing natural eliminative instincts and being unaware of the forces of nature and places and how they affect us are further causes of serious disease. Correct actions in the correct environment prevent disease.

The Gyu-zhi and Its "Tree of Health, Disease Diagnosis, and Treatment"

The *Gyu-zhi* (*rGyud-bzhi*) is the main medical text of Tibetan medical literature. It covers all aspects of disease, treatment and diagnosis and is said to contain all information necessary for recognizing and curing sickness. The version of the *Gyu-zhi* that is available today contains not only the original information brought from its original Indian source, but also the additional knowledge of Tibetan medicine drawn from other sources, like the pulse theory from China and herbal knowledge and urine analysis from native Tibet.

It contains four tantras or books, as has already been described, and these are altogether divided into one-hundred fifty-six chapters, a simple outline of which is found in the appendix to this book.

The First Tantra is the Root Tantra (*rTsa-rgyud*). It is the concise explanation of diseases and their examination. The Second is the Explication Tantra (*bShad-rgyud*) which explains in detail the doctrines of curing. The Third is the Pith Instruction Tantra (*Man-ngag-rgyud*). It details the treatment of specific diseases. It is the longest of the four tantras. The Fourth Tantra is the Last Tantra (*Phyi-ma'i-rgyud*). It integrates and sums up the first three.

The *Gyu-zhi* says that there are 404 diseases. This number is thought to be a reduction of the number 84,000—that being the number of diseases ascribed to each of the 84,000 obscurations (kleshas). One hundred and one divisions belong to the humors—42 to air, 26 to bile and 33 to phlegm. Three hundred and three other divisions are made. These are all described in the twelfth chapter, Second or Explication Tantra (*bShad-rgyud*).

In the First or Root Tantra there is given the theory of the human constitution, healthy and diseased, in terms of the simile of the Indian fig-tree. This provides a wonderful short descriptive summary of the entire medical system, and therefore an abbreviated version of it is presented here.[57]

This "Tree of Disease and Health" has three roots, nine trunks, forty-seven branches, two hundred and twenty-four leaves, two flowers and three fruits. The two flowers are health and long life. The three fruits are spiritual development, wealth, and happiness.

The roots and trunks are enumerated below; the branches and leaves are summarized.

I. DISEASE ROOT
A. *Balanced, Healthy Body Trunk*
1. Humors: air, bile, phlegm.
2. Constituents or supports: food (chyle), blood, flesh, fat, bone, marrow, semen.
3. Excretions: sweat, urine, feces.

B. *Imbalanced, Unhealthy Body Trunk*
1. Seeds of disease: three poisons—ignorance, lust and hate which cause phlegm, air, and bile.
2. Cause: season (hot or cold); evil spirits; wrong food; ill-conduct of life.
3. Entrance: skin, flesh, veins, bones, viscera.
4. Seat (proper places of the humors):
Phlegm in upper part of body;
Bile in middle part;
Wind in lower part.
5. Path:
Of wind—the bones, ears, skin, heart, "life-vein," large intestine;
Of bile—the blood, sweat, eyes, liver, small intestine;
Of phelgm—chyle, flesh, fat, marrow, semen, feces, urine, nose, tongue, lungs, spleen, kidney, stomach, bladder.
6. Rising Period:
Of wind—diseases of old people;
Of bile—diseases of adolescents and young adults;
Of phlegm—diseases of children.
Also in regard to place; also in regard to time and season.
7. Result or quality:
Wind—coarse, light, cold, etc.;
Phlegm—greasy, cool, heavy, etc.;
Bile—greasy, acute, hot, runny, etc.
8. Side Effect—Nine Fatal Diseases (causes thereof):
1. consumption of life span, karmic activity, or destiny;
2. disruption of bodily humors;
3. treatment goes similar to disease—disorder increases regardless of treatment;

4. wounds of vital organs;

5. exhaustion of life-wind, breath;

6. fever beyond treatment;

7. cold beyond treatment;

8. treatment cannot be sustained by body energy (can't tolerate medicine);

9. stealing of life by an evil spirit.

9. Abridgement: twelve causes by which any disease of the three humors is changed into a disease of another humor.

10. Disorders classified as hot or cold:

Wind and phlegm—cold, likened to water;

Bile and blood—hot, likened to fire;

Lymph and microorganisms—common to both hot and cold.

II. DIAGNOSTIC ROOT

A. *By sight*

1. Tongue:

Wind—dry, red, coarse, small red pimples on edge;

Bile—coated yellowish, bitter taste;

Phlegm—coated grey, sticky, soft, etc.

2. Urine:

Wind—thin, watery, big bubbles, bluish;

Bile—red, yellow, steamy, strong odor;

Phlegm—white, little steam and odor.

B. *By touch*

1. Pulses:

Wind—adrift ("like a melon floating on water, push down and it pops up"), empty—(you press and there is no beat), stops—(one out of seventy beats drops out on pressure);

Bile—tight, rapid, thin (stretched taut);

Phlegm—slow, sinks on pressure.

C. *By interrogation*

1. Wind disorders:

a. Cause—light and coarse food like Tibetan tea, pork and unripe food, behavior like grief;

b. Symptoms—

1. yawning, shivering

2. stretching limbs, sighing

3. ague—fever accompanied by chills and shivering

4. hip and joints ache
5. dry heaves
6. dulling of senses
7. irritation, mental agitation, giddiness
8. symptoms worse when hungry
9. insomnia, anxiety.

2. Bile disorders:
   a. Cause—sharp, acute, hot foods, violent conduct, sitting in hot sun or scorching heat;
   b. Symptoms—
   1. bitter taste in mouth
   2. severe headache
   3. intense body heat
   4. backache
   5. symptoms worse when digesting food.

3. Phlegm disorders:
   a. Cause—heavy, greasy food, sleeping in damp places;
   b. Symptoms—
   1. loss of appetite
   2. indigestion
   3. frequent vomiting
   4. loss of sense of taste
   5. distention of stomach
   6. frequent belching—smells of food eaten
   7. heaviness in mind and body, lazy
   8. coldness in body
   9. discomfort after eating.

III. TREATMENT ROOT

A. *Food and Beverage Trunk*

1. For Wind Disease:
   Food—horse, donkey, dried heavy meats that push down winds (greasy nutritious foods catch lightness of wind), seed oil, butter, brown sugar, garlic, onion;
   Beverage—hot milk, wine.

2. For Bile Disease:
   Food—curd, whey, fresh butter, wild animals, goat meat (is heavy and cold, increases wind and phlegm), dandelion, cool food;
   Beverage—luke-warm water, cool water from snow, boiled water cooled.

3. For Phlegm Disease:
Food—mutton, yak, animal organs, fish, honey, old barley, meat porridge, yak curd, hot food;
Beverage—old wine, boiling water, ginger soup.

B. *Behavior Trunk*
1. For Wind:
Relaxing in warm place with close friend—room with dark walls and friend who tells sweet stories; much sleep.
2. For Bile:
Stay in cool tranquil place—like being near sea in cool breezy place; behave in soft, gentle, relaxed slow manner.
3. For Phlegm:
Stay in the warm places, take exercise, sit near fire in warm bright room.

C. *Medicine Trunk*
1. Medicines in terms of tastes and powers:
a. For wind disorders: taste—sweet, sour, and saline; power—unctuous, heavy and soft;
b. For bile disorders: taste—sweet, bitter; power—thin, dull, blunt, cool;
c. For phlegm disorders: taste—hot, sour and acrid; power—sharp, rough, light.
2. Medicine in terms of types:
a. For wind—soups and medicine butter (a kind of syrup or paste);
b. For bile— decoctions (liquid infusions) and powders;
c. For phlegm—pills and powders.
3. Purging medicines:
a. For wind—suppositories, gentle enema medicants —3 kinds;
b. For bile—purgatives—4 kinds;
c. For phlegm—emetics—2 kinds;

D. *Physical Operations Trunk (98 kinds specifically mentioned)*
1. For wind:
Massage—smearing the body with (medicine) butter (and such oily applications) and moxibustion in the Mongolian manner.
2. For bile:
Phlebotomy and cool water therapies.
3. For phlegm:
Warm applications and cauterization and exercise.

Additional Notes on Diagnosis

It is said by Tibetan doctors that if one is unable, for whatever reasons, to rely on the twelve hundred ways of examining disease, then one can still rely with great accuracy upon the three basic ways: interrogation, sight, and touch. First the physician tries to establish, before he knows to which humor the disease belongs, whether it is a hot or cold disease, since all disease of the humors can be broken down into hot and cold disease. From knowing only that he can prescribe whole regimens of treatment.

In the initial interview involving interrogation, all sorts of facts about the patient's life are discussed and great importance is attached to the patient's sex life, which is discussed with some frankness. In spite of monastic celibacy (which is another matter entirely, often of sublimation related to tantric and yogic practice, especially that of holding the semen, thigle, and sending it back up the central column), the Tibetan people are hardly prudes. Tibetan medicine makes a direct connection between physical and mental well-being and a healthy sex life.

All the factors of behavior, diet, emotional and family life, and environment, as well as spiritual life, etc., are reviewed. On the basis

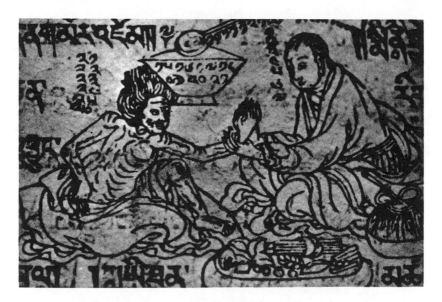

Figure 15 An illustration from a 17th century work by Sangye Gyatso, showing a Tibetan physician reading the pulse of a patient. The pulse is the main diagnostic tool of Tibetan medicine; it is also used for prognosis.

of this interrogation alone the doctor can determine much about disease. He is also checking the appearance of the patient: his radiance, manner, build, posture, speech, etc. There are twenty standard questions Tibetan doctors ask the patient during this interview, and these relate to the symptoms indicated on the "Tree of Health and Disease." After the interview, he proceeds to diagnosis by pulse and urine.

The Tibetans were famous for their urine analysis; it was their great indigenous contribution to Ayurvedic medicine. They can read it very, very well and believe urine reflects the internal state of the body like a mirror. For analysis, the urine is taken at the first passing in the morning. It is beaten, stirred, shaken, left to settle and even tasted for sweetness (for diabetes) by the doctor. He looks at its foam, sediment, color, steam, bubbles, smell, scum, etc. These are generally analyzed in terms of the humors, hot and cold disturbances, and the vital organs.

The *Gyu-zhi* describes normal or healthy urine as follows (from the second chapter of the Fourth Tantra):

> ...white with a yellowish tinge like the colour of freshly-melted butter; it is light, with a bad odour; the steam is normal and remains for a moderate time after the urine is passed; the bubbles in the urine are moderate in quantity; after the odour has disappeared, the sediment is blue with a yellowish tinge, neither thick nor thin; the scum is fine and settles around the edges of the container after the steam and the warmth of the urine have disappeared.[58]

Some remarks on the urine sediment in various diseases are as follows:

> If the sediment looks as though it could be picked up when settled, this signifies a disease of air; if it looks sprinkled it indicates a disease of cold; if it settles on the top this means a disease affecting the heart and lungs, if halfway it indicates diseases affecting the kidneys and intestines, etc.[59]

In regards to the pulse analysis, it is specified to a high degree and no doubt takes many years to perfect. It corresponds basically to the Chinese system. The left hand of the patient is examined by the right hand of the doctor and vice versa. As Dr. Yeshi Dhonden described it:

> The doctor feels the vessels with three fingers of both hands, index, middle and ring fingers.
>
> Within each of the three fingers, each half or side reads something different. This makes twelve analyses. With the right hand, the outside of the index finger (with the palm facing you) reads the heart; the inside of the index finger reads the intestines. The outside of the middle finger reads the spleen; the inside reads the stomach. The outside of the ring finger reads the left kidney; the inside reads the seminal vesicle or womb.
>
> With the left hand the outside of the index reads the lungs; the inside reads the large intestine. The outside of the middle finger reads the liver; the inside reads the gall bladder. The outside of the ring finger reads the right kidney; the inside reads the urinary bladder.[60]

In addition, pulsating veins are said to be of three types which are natural modes reflecting the nature of the individual. These are a female-vein type, male-vein type, and a neutral-vein type. It is said that there is a danger of mistaking the female pulse for a bile disease, the male pulse for a heat disorder, and the neutral pulse for a phelgm disease.

Regarding the theory of the elements—in Tibetan medicine they are connected with astrology, and astrology plays an important part in diagnosis and treatment of disease. Since the astrological aspects of the elements are derived from the Chinese system, these elements are sometimes known by their Chinese names: wood, fire, earth, iron and water.

The elements are connected with the seasons externally. This astrological and seasonal aspect is important in diagnosis. For example, if a doctor is examining a patient in spring, the element wood is strong; in summer, earth; autumn, iron; and in winter, water. Even if the doctor can't see the patient, Tibetans say he can know something about the condition of the disease just from astrological information about the patient. Then he can bring about harmony between the elements in the body, the disease, and the external world. So the predominance and nature of the elements becomes especially important in the growing and compounding of medicines.

In urine analysis and pulse diagnosis, astrological orientation is also important. In urine analysis, an astrological chart is used to mark

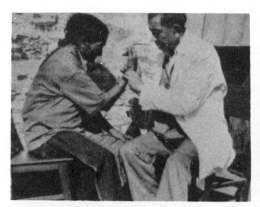
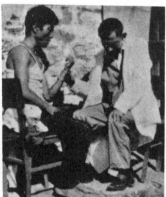
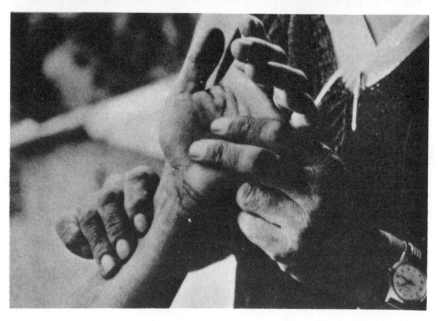

Figure 16 A modern Tibetan physician, Dr. Jampa Sonam of the Tibetan Medical Centre, checks patient's pulses (*A* and *B*) at a refugee settlement in South India. The exact finger placement (*C*) is important, as the pulse of the radial artery is considered the best informer on the condition of the body and is likened to ''a voice shouting across an open field in summer.''

off cardinal points on the container of urine. Each cardinal point and the four corners are identified with particular elements and the behavior of the urine in relation to these points indicates whether the disease can be treated and what its nature is. This astrological aspect of urine analysis is also part of a process of divination which will be detailed later in relation to invisible spirits.

Dying, Death and Rebirth

Death is, of course, an issue central to both religion and medicine. The *Gyu-zhi* devotes an entire chapter to the tokens of approaching death, and these include omens, dreams and physical symptoms.

In the Tibetan Buddhist view, the control of mind and the understanding of reality one has gained during life will determine one's ability to understand the experience of death and to control the course of consciousness there. The tradition holds that the purpose of doing Dharma practice is to be able to apply it at the moment of death.

The signs and stages of dying are recorded both in medical literature like the *Gyu-zhi* and in religious texts, particularly the terma of Guru Padmasambhava called *The Tibetan Book of the Dead (Bardo Thodol)*. According to the Tibetans, both in medical and religious theory, what happens during death is this. First, the five elements making up the physical body dissolve, and the consciousness is released into space. Second, one either recognizes the luminous nature of mind and reality as voidness or, if not, one experiences a variety of hallucinations and is directed by the force of karma into pleasant and unpleasant experiences (experienced with the mental body as being real—the way the mind experiences a dream) until one finally takes rebirth. In the womb, one has a variety of conscious experiences before birth.

The following description of what happens during the stages of death is based on material found in Chapter 7 of the Second Tantra of the *Gyu-zhi*, the *Tibetan Book of the Dead* and from teachings of H.H. Dudjom Rinpoche and Thinley Norbu Rinpoche.

The physical body is formed of the five inner elements corresponding to the five outer elements. Both the outer and the inner elements ultimately depend on and are generated from the absolute or secret elements inherent as essence in the wisdom mind or voidness. At death, the five inner elements supporting life dissolve and with them dissolve the five sense organs and the subtle energy centers or chakras. Also, the "karmic winds" overtake the five humoral winds at their seats in the body.

It is said that in order not to be afraid at the time of death when the dissolution of the elements occurs, one should know how to recognize the stages of their dissolving.

First, the element earth dissolves into water. Earth is located at the navel chakra, which falls apart. At this time the dying person loses strength and can't hold up his head, etc. The color of the complexion begins to fade. External forms cannot be clearly seen. Internally, the person feels a sinking into dullness and may ask to be lifted. The karmic force overtakes the "fire accompanying wind," and the body therefore cannot digest food; bodily warmth withdraws from the outer limbs toward the center of the body. The body feels heavy and hard to move.

Second, the water element dissolves into fire. Water is located at the subtle heart center, which falls apart. Externally, the nine orifices dry up, and there is the sensation of dryness and thirst. Internally, the mind becomes disturbed and angry. The karmic force overtakes the "life supporting wind" and mental powers are therefore disturbed.

Third, the fire element dissolves into wind. Fire is located in the throat center, which then falls apart. The person feels he is exhaling a cool breeze and it becomes hard to breathe. Internal warmth fades and he feels very cold. The mind becomes unfocused, spaced out. Sometimes there is awareness and sometimes not. The "downward clearing wind" becomes unbalanced and the person loses control of bodily functions like urination and defecation.

Fourth, wind dissolves into space. Wind is located at the lower "secret" genital center, which falls apart. There is no more inhalation, just the final exhalation. Now the mind becomes very disturbed and different experiences and hallucinations arise according to the dying person's past actions or karma. Aggressive people may feel they are being attacked by aggressive forces, and even though the person has no strength, he may try to repel the attackers. Peaceful people will have more peaceful visions. People who have done religious practice will have visions of the various deities coming to fetch them. The "pervasive wind" which circulates through the whole body is overtaken by the karmic winds and the body becomes stiff and rigid. When all the elements have thus dissolved into consciousness, the person feels he is being crushed under a huge weight.

Finally, consciousness dissolves into space. Consciousness is located at the forehead center, which falls apart. The breath completely stops. Internally, the "white father essence-drop" from the upper part of the head and the "red mother essence-drop" from the lower part of the body move toward the heart center. First there is an experience of white light like "a rising moon," then a flash of red light, then the consciousness and the "all pervading wind" become crowded in between the red and white essences and there is the experience of total darkness. At that moment, all the psychic channels (*rtsa*), forces (*rlung*), essences (*thig-le*) and consciousness dissolve into the heart center. And from the heart center, consciousness leaves the body and dissolves into space.

At this time of actual death it is like falling or fainting. After actual death has occurred, red and white fluids will discharge from the nostrils of the corpse. Until that happens, the person may appear to be dead but consciousness and the life-force have not yet left the body, and so the body should not be tampered with in any way. (This can take up to a few days for a normal person or a few weeks for advanced meditators, who benefit immensely from the unusual and powerful state of expanded consciousness at the time of dying.)*

The very moment when consciousness dissolves into space is crucial to Buddhist tantric practice, for space is revealed in that moment as brilliant luminosity, the clear light (the Dharmakaya). It is very important to remember the instructions at this time. Those who have practiced meditation and who have recognized the luminosity within will be able to mingle with this luminosity. This is called the "mother-child luminosity." At this point enlightenment can be reached.

The level of Dharma practice one has attained during life conditions the kind of death one experiences, and there are many kinds. The best practitioners mingle their consciousness with space as just described or they mingle into a rainbow.[61] Intermediate practitioners may just go like a "child" or "beggar" without any grasping or clinging.

---

*In cases where the body has been very badly damaged by disease, the fluids may not discharge from the nose (and/or sexual organs).

Ordinary practitioners can practice "pho-wa," the transference of consciousness out the top of the head to the Buddha-field of their choice, where they will await rebirth in the presence of the Buddhas and will receive teachings.

It is said to be extremely important for all persons that the consciousness leave the body by exiting upward through the central channel and out of the top of the head through the soft spot on the skull—called the "Gate of Brahma." To exit out of the lower centers is said to start a course toward lower rebirth.

According to Tibetan medicine, then, it is important that the dying person not be under the influence of strong drugs and pain killers which impair his ability to recognize the stages of dying and especially his ability to recognize the clear light. Furthermore, such mind altering drugs will affect the consciousness in the realms between death and rebirth if enlightenment is not reached at the moment of death.

The stages in between death and rebirth are vividly described in the *Tibetan Book of the Dead*. This book is meant to be read aloud to the dying and dead person. Basically, it identifies the progressive states of the visions in the realm between death and rebirth (the intermediate state called the *bar-do*) and exhorts the dead person to recognize that all he is experiencing is a projection of his own mind. For if this is recognized at any point, the consciousness can become enlightened. However, it becomes progressively harder to realize this during the stages in the bardo, it being easiest to recognize in the initial flash of clear light. But even partial recognition and remembrance that all one is experiencing is a projection of mind will help assuage the terror and turbulent emotions that the consciousness is experiencing. For even though there is no material body, the consciousness feels a whole range of sensations and emotions and sees a whole world of forms and visions just as he does during a dream with the dream body. What one experiences in the stages of the bardo is conditioned by one's karma, the mental habits one has developed during life, and one's last dying thoughts.

The *Tibetan Book of the Dead* is a most extraordinary piece of literature. As Dr. Carl Jung wrote in his "Psychological Commentary" on it, "For years, ever since it was published, the *Bardo Thodol* has been my constant companion, and I owe to it not only many stimulating ideas and discoveries but also many fundamental insights. . . . The Bardo Thodol offers one an intelligible philosophy addressed to human beings rather than to gods or primative savages. Its philosophy contains the quintessence of Buddhist psychological criticism; and, as such, one can truly say that it is of an unexampled superiority."[62]

At the end of the journey through the intermediate regions of the bardo, the consciousness takes rebirth. Tibetan medicine says there are four types of birth: by moisture, by egg, by womb, and by spontaneous manifestation. The latter is a mental birth of two types: superior and inferior. In the superior type, enlightened beings can take birth on objects like a lotus or by entering into various inanimate object forms (like a bridge, etc.) in order to help sentient beings. In the inferior type, a being may be suddenly reborn in a hell realm, for example.

Enlightened beings and bodhisattvas can direct the force of their consciousness in the bardo and take conscious rebirth in ways appropriate for helping other beings. Thus, Tibetan lamas sometimes predict where they will be reborn before they die; as children they are recognized as the tulku or the emanation body of the previous incarnation. They show signs of remembering their previous life. For example, the lineage of the Dalai Lamas is recognized in this way. And this is how the great lamas can trace their incarnations back through the centuries, and how they continue various lineages of teaching and transmission.

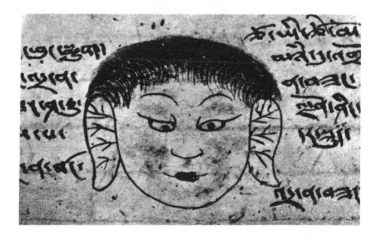

Figure 17 Pediatrics is one of the eight branches of Tibetan medicine. This picture, from a handwritten manuscript, illustrates a diagnostic technique of examining ears, since children's diseases, it is said, cannot be diagnosed through the pulse.

For ordinary beings to take human birth, the karmic mind-stream of consciousness in the bardo must be drawn back into the world by seeing two human beings in the act of copulation. Only those beings or mind-streams with residue karma with particular parents can find a womb to enter. The rest are said to continue to wander around waiting to find a proper womb.

When the mind sees the two parents in the act of making love, it feels attraction to one parent and aversion towards the other. This is the essential feeling that must arise. This is described in the *Gyu-zhi*:

> Three things are needed for the formation of a body: perfect semen without any flaw caused by disease, menstrual blood [by which the Tibetans imply the egg], and the mind of the intermediate (bardo) state driven by the right karma. The nature of all the five elements is necessary for its continued existence: this is the cause of conception. It depends on the linkings of the mind whether its body is going to become male or female. If it identifies itself with the semen and is attracted by the mother and dislikes the father, it is going to be born as a boy. If it identifies itself with the mother's menstrual blood, which must be in its right time and flawless, and if anger is felt with the mother, then a girl is going to be born.[63]

The consciousness being attracted to the sexual organ of one parent, anger arises toward the other parent, and this arising of anger creates cessation of the bardo existence. A brief death experience is gone through, seeing the clear light etc., then at the moment of conception the reincarnating consciousness merges with the mixture of sperm and ovum and fades into unconsciousness. With the support of the five elements, the particles become thoroughly mixed and the embryo comes into being. The psychic channels and chakras are formed by the eighth week, the life vein and the navel chakra being the first of these, and from them the body develops. The weekly stages of the development of the embryo are described in detail in the second chapter of the Second Tantra of the *Gyu-zhi*.

Gradually consciousness returns to the embryo, and during the sixth month the embryo begins to have emotions such as happiness or sadness. During the twenty-sixth week it is said to be able to remember its former lives.

In *The Jewel Ornament of Liberation* by the eleventh century Tibetan philosopher-doctor-saint, Gampopa, the misery a being experiences in the womb is described in greater detail than in the *Gyu-zhi*. For example, Gampopa says, "When a mother keeps an unbalanced diet by giving preference to cold food, the embryo suffers the pain of a naked person being thrown upon ice. In the same way there is pain when the food is either too hot or too sour. When too much is taken it is as if you are crushed between rocks; when too little, it is as if you were suspended and rocked in mid-air. . . . When a mother indulges too often in sexual intercourse during her pregnancy, the embryo feels as if it were beaten with thorns." During the thirty-seventh week, he says, "the consciousness of the foetus, grieved by the state of dirtiness, stench, darkness, and imprisonment, conceives the idea of escaping."[64]

The pain the baby feels as it is being born is also described as an excruciating trauma: "At birth it feels like a cow that is flayed alive and as if stung by a wasp, and when it is bathed the touch of warm water gives it a feeling as if it was beaten."[65]

All births are not, perhaps, necessarily so distressing—Gampopa is illustrating here the inescapability of suffering in life, death, the bardo, and birth. As for pregnancy and childbirth, Tibetan medicine has its own detailed system and even a form of birth control pill. There are medicines given at the time of birth to relax the muscles and make delivery easier—a medicine butter that is both eaten and rubbed onto the vagina, also medicines given during pregnancy and after delivery.

During pregnancy, the importance of a loving psychic relationship between mother and fetus is emphasized, and the fetus is treated as a conscious individual. And after birth, in infancy and childhood, the new being exhibits distinct habits and dispositions due to its own inherited karma from former lives.

7

Somatic Medicine: Curative Aspects

The functional genius of Tibetan medicine is expressed through its actual ability to effect cures, the practical application of its elaborate medical, mystical, and philosophical theory.

Substances from which medicines are made, materia medica, abounded in Tibet. The high altitude and cold climate of the Himalayan plateaus seemed to have imparted to its growing things a specialness appropriate to the "Rooftop of the World." The presence of special curative herbs is one of the few things we know about the culture of shamanic pre-Buddhist Tibet. It is said that the earliest fathers of Chinese medicine, Emperors Shen Nung and Huang Ti, knew of the wonders of Tibetan herbs and described them in the *Pents'ao* and *Nei Ching* respectively. Tibetan doctors purportedly had over a thousand natural substances from which they could compound medicines.

In Tibetan medicines, it is not so much the presence of one particular ingredient but the particular combination of many ingredients that provides the desired therapeutic effect. In treating an ebullition of a humor, a swelling up of air for example, the medicine has to reduce that over-abundance of the humor and also treat any secondary humoral disturbances that the primary ebullition has created. That secondary ebullition may appear as the obvious symptom: a phlegm disturbance in the stomach may actually be

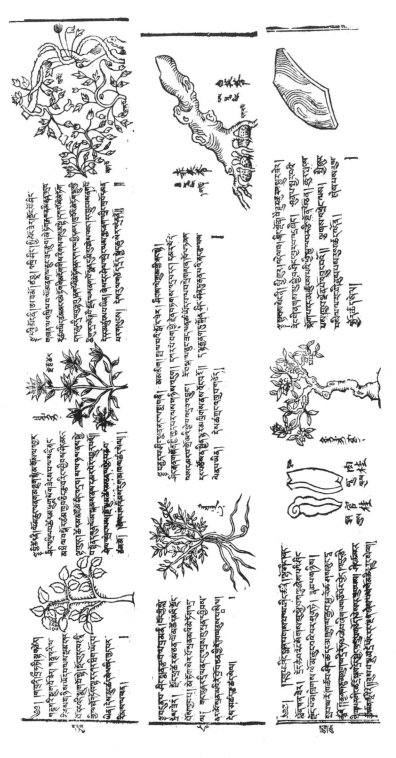

Figure 18 Medicinal substances from trees, as seen in *An Illustrated Tibeto-Mongolian Materia Medica of Ayurveda.* The first tree is brown ga-bra, whose trunk is "spotted white as though spattered with yogurt." The fresh twig is used to treat infectious fevers caused by wind (*rlung*).

caused by too much air there, which has slowed down the digestive process thus creating a blockage and excess of phlegm.

In that case, the doctor may first give emetics to clear the phlegm, and this after he has thoroughly prepared the patient for the emetic by giving him various loosening substances. After that, he will treat the overabundance of air with a preparation especially suited to the particular kind and location of air disturbance. The medicine may also contain ingredients which prevent further humoral disharmony which might arise from use of medicine. For example, ginger or long pepper are often added to anti-air preparations in order to insure that a disturbance of bile is not aggravated by the medicine itself.

The patient's psychological, emotional and spiritual make-up are also factors which must be considered in the making of medicine— even in completely non-psychiatric cases. Such factors are understood in terms of their physical repercussions. Therefore medicines must be compounded with an eye towards inhibiting certain spiritual-emotional factors that have affected the arising of the sickness. This is another instance of how even the most practical giving of medicines is actually a very holistic, individualized treatment of the whole person, no factor in isolation.

Tibetan Pharmacology

There are numerous Tibetan medical texts dealing with their vast pharmacopeia and describing the substances in various aspects and in depth, but not one of them has been translated into English.

Information about the action and effects of medicines is also found scattered throughout most medical texts. The Second Tantra of the *Gyu-zhi* provides much specific information about the qualities and actions of medicinal substances—all within the subject of general medicine. One looks forward to the time when the specifically pharmacological texts are in translation.

Some idea of the extent of the Tibetan pharmacopoeia can be gained from the book *The Illustrated Tibetan Mongolian Materia Medica of Ayurveda* (in Tibetan, edited by Prof. Dr. Lokesh Chandra), which lists nearly seven hundred medicinal substances obtained from minerals, plants and animals. These are presented in various categories, which are translated into English in the Table of Contents. They are as follows:

    I. Gems and Metals (a. precious substances which can't be melted; b. precious substances which can be melted).

II. Substances derived from rocks and minerals (a. meltable; b. not meltable).

III. Medicinal earths (natural; manufactured; salts).

IV. Exudates and secretions.

V. Medicinal substances obtained from trees (fruits and nuts; blossoms; leaves; twigs; stalks; roots; saps).

VI. Medicinal substances obtained from boiled extracts of various parts of plants.

VII. Medicinal plants, herbs, and grasses (roots; leaves; flowers; fruits; leaves-stalks-flowers-fruits together; entire plant; cultivated plants, i.e., bearded; leguminous, and roots).

VIII. Medicines obtained from sentient creatures (birds; herbivores; wild animals; magical birds; domestic animals; those living in holes and burrows; those thriving in moisture).

The pharmacopeia of Tibet is even larger than that of Chinese medicine and includes plants and medicines which were not originally native to Tibetan soil. But in actual fact and practice Tibetan doctors, like their Chinese counterparts, normally select from a much smaller range of substances.

An excellent overview of Tibetan medical pharmacology is found in the medicine mandala. In the four directions of the mandala grow four divisions of nature that provide a fundamental diagram of herbal pharmacology.

The four medicine mountains of the mandala provide treatment for hot diseases; cold diseases; all diseases; and maintenance of the six vital functions and organs. These four divisions of medicine, which can be further reduced to two, preventative and curative, are a miniature model of the larger medical system.

The external or "outer" medicine mandala is, in seed form, a map of the integral relationships between diseases, pharmacology, and the other qualities of being associated with the directions of any mandala (see chart on chakras and information on Five Buddhas).

The medicinal plants of the medicine mountains in the four quarters of the medicine mandala are said to have been planted by the beautiful Yitogma, an emanation of the medicine goddess Nectar Mother.

In the East is the "Fragrant Mountain" Ponadan. Here in a mild climate grow a jungle of medicine plants that can be smelled from miles away, a forest of myrobalan (*Terminalia chebula*, Tib. *a-ru-ra*), the "supreme medicine." This is what the Medicine Buddha holds in his hand. Different parts of the tree, especially the fruit and stem, are used for a multitude of diseases.

Myrobalan is good for fevers and colds. The root is good for bone diseases, the trunk for flesh, the branch for nerve disorders and sinew, the bark for skin, the leaf for diseases of the "hollow organs," the flower for sense organs, and the fruit for heart and the solid organs. Myrobalan has all the six tastes and all the eight powers of Tibetan medicine. Its perfume drives away all four hundred and four diseases.

In the West is the "Cool Mountain" called Malaya. Here grow the "Six Good Things" (*bzang-drug*), the six fabulous medicines for maintenance of the body. They are: nutmeg for wind; clove for the life vein (at the heart); cubeb for the spleen; cardamon for the kidney; saffron for the liver; and bamboo pith for the lungs. These are said simply to give happiness to people.

In the rocky parts of the mountain are found five kinds of pitch—gold, silver, copper, iron, and lead—which are good for fevers. Five kinds of quartz are also there, and five kinds of medicinal hot springs. The springs coming from coal are good for fever; from coal and sulphur for cold diseases and disordered fluids; from coal and pitch for bile diseases, etc. In Tibet there are many kinds of hot springs and the Tibetan medical use of thermal springs was an entirely indigenous development.

On the cliffs are medicinal stones like turquoise, as well as various salts. The forest is filled with fragrant scents and with the sweet songs of birds. There are peacocks, elephants (their gall stone is good for fever), bears (their bile is for liver disorders), and musk deer (musk counteracts sepsis and worm diseases). As for turquoise, it is said to help in every illness and thus to promote long life. It is especially useful in counteracting food poisoning and liver disorders.

In the North is Gangchen, the "Snowclad Mountain." It has the nature of the moon and the quality of cold. Here grow medicines that combat all hot diseases. Here are white sandalwood, camphor, aloeswood and margosa. They are bitter, sweet, astringent and bland. Their perfume lowers temperatures.

In the South is Begche, the "Thunderbolt Mountain." It has the nature of sun and the quality of heat. Here grow medicine plants with hot power. They combat cold diseases. They are red sandalwood, pomegranate, black pepper and long pepper. They are hot, sour, and salty. Their perfume normalizes imbalance of cold.

Qualities of Medicinal Substances

Medicine plants all share specific qualities and the nature of the five elements which produce them: "Earth forms the base; water moistens them; fire generates heat and growth; air causes movement assisting growth; and sky allows space for growth." Each medicine plant, however, is affected by the predominance of elements where it grows. These elements are coordinated with tastes as follows:

> Where earth and water predominate, sweet taste results.
> Where fire and earth predominate, sour taste results.
> Where water and fire predominate, salty taste results.
> Where water and air predominate, bitter taste results.
> Where fire and air predominate, acrid taste results.
> Where earth and air predominate, astringent taste results.[66]

Therefore, the same species of a medicine plant may be quite different in effect depending on the conditions of its growth. The manner, time, and season of their being picked and prepared also affects their action. Tibetan doctors pay great attention to these and other subtle factors influencing medicinal substances. Such factors may in part explain why medicinal substances of non-Western cultures, when tested in the West, often fail to show the qualties which they are known for in their own environment. This also brings up the question of classifications of medical plants—for the major works on plants of the East do not make distinctions along these lines. At any rate, we again have another example of subtle and spiritual factors, this time those of the environment mixing with simple, basic and substantial aspects of Tibetan medicine—the medicine plants themselves.

Each element predominating in the medicinal substance has specific healing qualities. The qualities of the medicinal substances having the nature of one specific element are formulated as follows (according to the *Gyu-zhi*):[67]

> *Earth*—heavy, strong, firm, and pungent; these produce energy and combat air diseases.
> *Water*—cool, heavy, smooth and soft; these oil, moisten and smooth the system and combat bile diseases.
> *Fire*—sharp, hot, light and rough; produce warmth in body, strengthen the seven constituents, enrich the complexion and combat phlegm diseases.

Air—light, unstable, cold, and rough; give strength to body, facilitate bodily movements and the distribution of nutrition and combat diseases of phlegm combined with bile.

Space/Sky—hollow; they combat diseases of bile, phlegm and air. All plants and substances have the nature of sky, but some plants are are chiefly sky nature.

Medicines are also classified according to taste. Saffron, meat, butter and honey are sweet, for example. Pomegranate, curd and yeast are sour. Gentian, musk and aconite are bitter. Long pepper, ginger and garlic are acrid. Myrobalan is astringent.

In addition to taste, substances are classed according to inherent powers and secondary qualities; the former never change, but the latter can. For example, according to Dr. Yeshi Dhonden, raw brown sugar has the power of heaviness and the quality of warmth, and in this state it is used to combat wind ailments. When sugar is refined, however, its warmth changes to coolness, and as such it is no longer helpful for wind disorders.

According to the *Gyu-zhi,* medicines can be prepared from every substance on earth. The idea that every substance on earth has a medicinal property because it shares in the nature of the elements is illustrated in a story of Atreya and Jivaka.

When Jivaka was studying medicine under Atreya at Taxila, Atreya sent him and the other students to find a substance that could not be used for healing. All the other students returned carrying different plants and matter, but only Jivaka came back empty-handed. This showed the thoroughness of Jivaka's knowledge, that he fully realized that everything has medicinal qualities.

Medicine-Making and State of Mind

Medicinal substances are venerated for their healing powers. A good Tibetan doctor will treat them with due respect and regard them as an offering to the Medicine Buddha.

The main thing is that one should not make medicine without utter and complete devotion to the guru and to the Medicine Buddhas. Without demonstrating devotion of this kind, one will not even be able to receive medicine teachings. Tibetan doctors are not interested in telling their secrets or convincing anyone. They are interested in maintaining a pure samaya with the Medicine Buddha, for from that comes all medicine power.

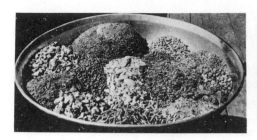
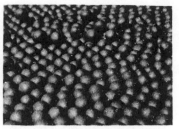

Figure 19 Twenty-five dried herbal ingredients (left) for a particular medicine formula. The substances go through many stages of preparation to make the final pills (right).

From the very moment a doctor goes to gather medicine substances, he is aware that his state of mind adds a crucial factor to the effectiveness of the medicine. When he gathers the plants, he is not only aware of conditions of soil and sunlight and how these affect the predominating element of each plant, but he is also regarding himself as the Medicine Buddha and the substances he is collecting as the medicine mandala. His sensitivity and clarity of mind, and especially his purity of intention to help others, render him more or less capable of making good medicine.

Instructions for making medicines are usually cryptically stated in medical texts. Much is left unsaid—the doctor is supposed to know the full implications. After a doctor has gathered and dried the substances, they will be cleaned and possibly detoxified. Then they will be measured out according to whatever ratio has been indicated in the texts.

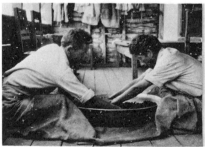
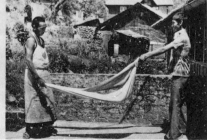

Figure 20 A stage in the process of making a pill (left); here the formula is being kneaded. A lama and a layman (right) with a medicinal substance in the final stages of the sun-drying process, outside the Medical Centre in Dharamsala.

While the doctor cleans and measures the ingredients, he must maintain mindfulness. Thus his handling of the medicines is often very beautiful and graceful; in this way the mere arranging of ingredients on a plate or tray becomes the making of a mandala, a precise ritual evocative of profound awareness. The ingredients are then chopped or ground up as the text indicates.

The actual compounding and preparation of medicine brings into play the spiritual development of the doctor along with his medical knowledge. All making of medicine begins with a prayer. The doctor must keep an absolutely pure mind and handle all substances, whether they be cat feces or lotus flowers, with equal respect. Nothing is thought of as vile. No matter how long or laborious the task, the doctor must keep a good attitude and never feel bored or inject any negative thoughts or emotions into the process—those being highly destructive and poisonous.

There must be no break in the process of making a medicine. Once it has started, it has to be continuous, no matter how many days it might take (for example, it takes at least three days to purify mercury). A break in the process will cause the medicine to lose its power.

With the right wisdom and skillful means, everything can become medicine, as the story of Atreya and Jivaka shows. Because all things proceed from mind, because of the essential identity of the elemental substance of manifest existence, because "all partake of the nature of the self-existing equanimity," all things are interrelated. All things can be used to rebalance and reharmonize the imbalance of illness.

Medicines and Other Treatments

The most popular ways of giving medicines are the gentle methods (*'jam-pa che*). These include burning and inhaling incense— very important in psychiatry and air disturbances. The incenses are compounded of many different herbs and ingredients.

There are also special herbal baths, one of which is five herbal grasses added to bath water for medicinal soaking. Tibetan doctors prescribe the use of the wonderful Tibetan hot springs in a variety of ways as water therapy. Medicine oils and butters are used for massaging and annointing the body. These medicine butters (*sman-mar*) are highly thought of. The older the butter, the more effective.

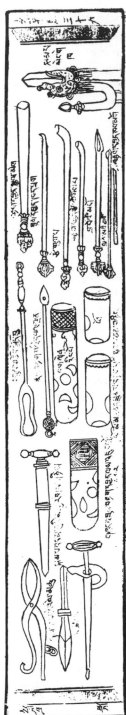
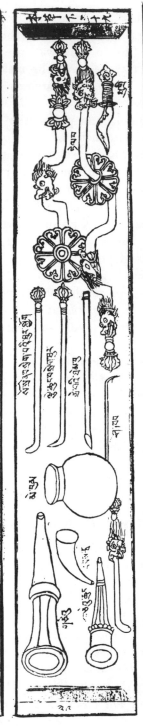
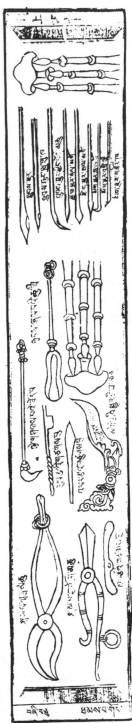

Figure 21 Tibetan surgical instruments. Minor surgery was performed in Tibet, but generally only as a last resort.

This is because the elements in the butter are thought to become stronger with aging.

There are stronger methods (*rtsub che*) of treatment. These include bloodletting, lancing, moxibustion and acupuncture. Acupuncture and moxibustion are done with restraint, and fewer points are used than in the Chinese system. Special herbal mixtures for moxibustion are burned on major points which are the same for acupuncture (the ones used for mental disorders are described later in the notes following the psychiatric texts).

The straightforward administration of medicine mixtures (herbal, mineral, etc.) forms a separate category. These medicines may be made as pills, decoctions (*thang-sman,* the boiling down of essences), powders, syrups, oils and butters (here for ingesting not rubbing), ash-like medicines (*thal-sman*), concentrated medicines (*khan-da*) and wines.

Medicines are taken with or coated with certain substances—medicine vehicles. They are boiled water, alcohol (usually the Tibetan beer known as "chang"), sugar, treacle, and honey. The effects of the medicine ingredients are said to vary according to the vehicle.

The most fundamental and favored type of treatment in Tibetan medicine is modification of behavioral and dietary patterns; this is the most gentle manner of therapy and always the first to be relied upon. Other catagories of treatment include cleansing procedures such as emetics, which can be therapeutic in themselves or preparatory to the administration of other medicaments.

The last classification of healing methods is known as violent or radical (*drag-po che*). It includes minor surgery and cauterization and is avoided unless absolutely necessary. As for major surgery, it was supposedly practiced in early times in Tibet, but in the wake of a failed heart operation on the mother of a ninth century king, it was outlawed and mostly abandoned.

Part II

Tibetan Medical Psychiatry

May those who find themselves in trackless,
    fearful wildernesses—
The children, the aged, the unprotected,
Those stupified and the insane—
Be guarded by beneficent celestials.

                —from Shantideva's
                  Bodhicharyavatara

8

Medical Psychiatry

All the major emphases of the Tibetan Buddhist world view meet in its psychiatric tradition. Psychiatric theory, diagnosis and treatment are inextricably bound up with the three types of Tibetan medicine: Dharmic, tantric and somatic. Varied aspects of these three remedial approaches come into play in any one psychiatric case. Ritual exorcism, mantras and other religious practice, change of diet and environment, acupuncture and most especially herbal medicines make up the treatment program.

The psychiatric tradition which we are about to detail does not include the psychiatric disorders of children or the aged. Both child psychiatry and geriatrics are separate divisions within the medical tradition. Chapter 73 of the Third Tantra of the *Gyu-zhi* lists fifteen spirits which are thought to attack young children and cause nervous disorders in them. Children are said to be highly susceptible to invasion by negative forces and we are advised to protect them from that possibility as much as we can. For example, one is never supposed to startle a youngster for it is exactly in such a moment of suspended consciousness, as in a trance due to fear, that the invading force can enter; this can also happen when the child is sleeping.

Geriatrics is one of the eight main divisions of Tibetan medicine.[1] It is mostly concerned with rejuvenation and the use of special medicines to slow the aging process and revitalize the mind and body. Much attention is paid to ginseng. No translations of any geriatric texts or the specific geriatrics chapter of the *Gyu-zhi* have yet been made.

Before we detail the adult medical psychiatry of Tibet it seems useful to review the three separate approaches to madness that have emerged in the history of psychiatry as they relate to the Tibetan system which is unusual in interweaving them so consciously.

Magical-Religious Approach: From the time of earliest human cultures, pathological disturbances of mind and spirit have lent themselves to religious interpretations. Theories of possession by evil spirits have been documented in almost all primitive, tribal and shamanic cultures. This view is also held by the great world religions. It seems to be an archaic shared belief, a natural way of understanding some of the mysterious pathological disorders of personality and behavior which characterize mental disease.

Possession by evil spirits is the oldest "pre-rational" medical theory. In the Hindu Vedic period, millennia before traditional Ayurvedic medicine developed, the term *bhuta-vidya* was used to designate all diseases (not just mental) caused by invisible forces. *Bhuta-vidya* later became the name of the fourth branch of classical Ayurveda, psychiatry and neuropathology, which covered diseases caused by spirits, including epilepsy and leprosy and mental illness.

In the Tibetan psychiatric tradition possession by evil spirits is a major cause of insanity. Treatment in this magico-religious aspect includes tantric and yogic practices of healing ("magic") as well as the practice and application of Dharma (religion). As far as "magic" is concerned, nowhere was it more highly developed than in Tibet. The country was always known as a land of magic and magicians, a mysterious place where monks had enormous psychic and spiritual powers. Tibet even became a symbol of the occult. For many centuries the "magic" of Tibet was misunderstood and thought to be heinous heathen necromancy, witchcraft and general bedevilment not fit to be called religion and certainly not medicine.

Fortunately, this misunderstanding of Tibetan Buddhism is no longer prevalent. Upon examining even the most elaborate rituals for exorcism of evil forces one finds that the essence of Dharma is at the heart of these "magical" practices—in the form of compassion and the commitment to the well-being of others.

In the religious approach to healing mental illness different Dharma practices are applied as medicine. It should be noted here that when one speaks of the medicine of Dharma what is meant is not just the traditional form and practice of orthodox Buddhism (although of course it can mean that) but the heroic effort to progress spiritually out of unconsciousness and into full awareness. One meaning of the

Sanskrit word *dharma* is that which holds one on the path, the path of truth and insight. The Tibetan word for Dharma, which is *chos,* comes from the verb *'chos,* which means to cure or to heal. This serves to underscore the medical analogy: the practice of Dharma is the means for remedying the mental and emotional obscurations that produce all harm and prevent enlightenment.

Organic Approach: The organic approach to psychopathology in Tibetan medicine is grounded in the humoral theory—the "rational" science of medicine. The three humors have associated psychological dispositions which can, by various causes of humoral imbalance, express themselves as psychopathological disorders. Further, the psychiatric aberrations of phlegm, bile and wind often include related physical disorders.

Of course the Dharma is at the heart of this approach also because it is never forgotten that basic confusion (ignorance, unawareness) generated the defilements of aversion and craving and caused the three humors to arise on the organic plane in the first place.

This relationship between the three humors and the three primary mental defilements expresses the basic psychosomatic theory of Tibetan medicine and psychiatry. Different treatments and medicines are applied to influence the mind through the body.

All this implies that Tibetan medicine presupposes that emotions have physiological functions, perhaps like the biochemical correlates of emotions that modern science is discovering. Further, that the substances used in Tibetan psychiatric medicine are said to have the composition (in terms of elements, tastes, etc.) that is deficient in the disorder they remedy also echos the latest research findings—the psychoactive drugs mimic the body's own neurochemistry.

Psychological Approach: The three defilements that generated the humors are also the three types of psychological forces that precipitate psychiatric humoral imbalances. Too much confusion, hatred, or desire causes psychiatric disturbances. The whole psychological approach to psychopathology is based on Dharma in this way, for the essence of the arising of all conditioned existence is the development of self-centered ego and its subsequent obscurations of mind.

On a more relative and immediate level, psychological disturbances are understood to originate from such causes as emotional strain and mental pressure, stress, problems of love, family relations, loss of possessions, status and loved ones, isolation, pressure, anxiety, overwork. All these are classified in Tibetan medical psychiatry as factors which cause the "mind to go off" in various ways.

Dharma is not only the basis of the theory of the nature of mind, it is also a preventative medicine for mental sickness. It builds a strong mind that cannot be easily over-powered by emotional strains, intellectual pressures or even evil spirits. As one Tibetan doctor said in illustration of this, "When people, for example, lose their country [like the Tibetans have] they become too sad and full of grief, and they sometimes begin to lose their senses. But by practicing Dharma they can remember it is not only they who suffer. Everywhere people suffer the same."[2] This is a rather poignant illustration of how the medicine of Dharma can turn intense suffering into compassion and wisdom rather than into self-pity and insanity.

Mind's Primary Relationship to the Winds (Airs, rLung)

Of the three humors, wind is the one primarily associated with mental disturbances. This is a basic Ayurvedic theory. In the classical Ayurvedic tradition, one of the principal terms for madness was *vatula,* literally "inflated with wind," and this indicates the central connection. Wind is the humor primarily associated with mind and mental derangements. The relationship between life and mind and breath—the life energy (*prana*) within the breath and the breath's direct effect (through its control) on mind—is one of the most important and central aspects of Indian thought and yogic practice.

Wind is the subtlest of the humors and the one most like mind. By stabilizing the gross winds and the subtle wind (with its inherent life force) through yogic practice, the mind also becomes stabilized.

Most psychiatric cases are understood to have disturbed air, and most grave disturbances of air are thought to lead to mental instability and depression. In fact, intense neurotic behavior and the psychological and physiological symptoms of nervousness are called simply the disease "sok-lung" (Tib. *srog-rlung*), a disorder of life-wind.

All the winds circulate as energy currents in numerous channels and pathways (*rtsa*) of the body, but the most subtle part of the "life-bearing wind" remains without moving inside the life-vein which is connected to the heart. This very subtle life-force, the sok-lung *(srog-rlung),* is the main support of consciousness.

As Garma C.C. Chang explained, "Mind and prana [*rlung,* psychic energy] are two facets of one entity—they should never be treated as two separate things. Mind is that which is aware; prana is the active energy which gives support to this awareness.''[3] Although consciousness (and the life-force) is spread throughout the body, the "owner" of it is the very subtle life-force in the life-vein at the heart.

This life-vein (*srog-rtsa*) most likely corresponds to the vagus nerve, although some have identified it with the aorta; it may, in fact, be neither of these. One part of it is said to run between the lungs and the heart (wherein moves the "life-bearing wind") and another between the heart and the brain, branching off into smaller channels to the various sense organs (the "pervasive wind" moves in this part).

Consciousness becomes disturbed and even insane when the inner winds, for various reasons, circulate in ways and places they shouldn't. Specifically, they inflate the vital channel and insert at the part in the heart where the subtle life-force dwells.

When this happens, the mind power of the individual begins to disintegrate and hallucinations and all sorts of distortions in perception of reality arise. The heart itself (*snying*) is synonymous with mind in the Tibetan system; this is because consciousness, mental clarity and sense of self-identity arise from the heart center. Sensory input is carried by the all-pervasive wind through the nerves or channels to the brain, where it is registered, but the consciousness relating to sensory impressions and thoughts resides in the heart.

The consciousness at the heart is supported by the most subtle life-force there, and that life-force can be disturbed by the humoral winds as described above. This can happen in many ways, both psychological and physical. For example, sudden extreme anger carried by the "pervasive wind" swells the currents travelling in the life vein, pressuring the most subtle life-wind out of place and into the heart; it is this disturbance that causes consciousness to become distorted.

All the winds are interconnected. So, for example, by withholding the need to urinate, the wind that controls urination is disturbed, and this can lead to disturbance of the very subtle life-wind at the heart. Additionally, physical causes not directly related to the winds, for example, malfunctions of the humors bile or phlegm (or whatever adversely affects the condition of the channels—since the relationship is that the channels support the winds and winds support the mind), can alter the state of consciousness at the heart.

It should also be noted here that the results of disturbing the life-force at the heart are not only psychological but also physical. Wind in the heart produces stress disorders like high blood pressure and other cardiovascular diseases.

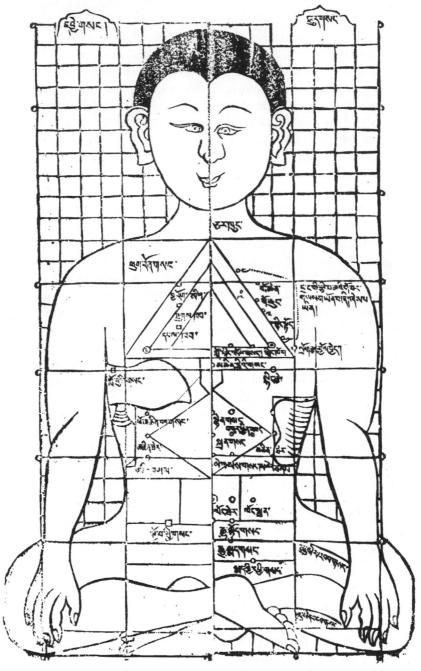

Figure 22 The front half of a medical chart from *An Illustrated Tibeto-Mongolian Materia Medica* (it is actually two folios aligned together). It shows the location of the "secret" points used to treat various diseases through moxibustion, acupuncture, etc. The triangle in the chest describes the heart center where the control of consciousness is said to reside. Just above the corner of the triangle on the viewer's right is the point for "madness made by the life-vein."

Generally, the disorder known as "wind," "life-wind" or "heart-wind" is brought on by worry, strain, overwork, sorrow, anger, sudden shock or fear, etc. and manifests psychologically in its early stages as over-sensitivity, anxiety, and emotional instability. Physiologically there is quickened heart beat, dizziness, insomnia, loss of appetite, lack of co-ordination, and accident proneness—because of the disturbed energy currents inside the body. Another physical sign is a crack down the middle of the tongue. There is a constant cycle between elation and depression, continuous quick changes back and forth in mood. If left untreated, it can develop into psychosis.

When the very subtle life-force supporting consciousness is out of place, then the consciousness which the person experiences feels "wrong" or "alien," which could give rise to the sense of being possessed by an outside force. Also, from the point of view of demonic possession, the demons are said to enter through various channels and make their way to the heart where they take over consciousness. In this sense, they act exactly like emotions.

In the yogic and tantric systems, one speaks of consciousness and the life-force thigle which reside in the heart center and central channel, rather than in the organ of the heart and the life-vein. However, the tantric and medical systems are parallel and related in certain specifics. For one thing, the heart or heart-center is what connects the physical and subtle bodies. For another, the tantric system accepts the five divisions of wind-energies described in the medical system but speaks of all the winds being driven by mental-emotional obscurations of the karmic force (thus called the karmic winds) and of having inherent within them the wisdom wind or "yeshe-lung." These winds circulate in numerous subtle channels and physical pathways, which can be reduced to the three main subtle channels and the five main channels of consciousness.

The subtle channels are made of light; they are not substantial but are part of the energetic sub-structure of the physical body. What is rather confusing is that the Tibetans use the same word—*rtsa*—for the physical veins and nerves and for the subtle channels.

The five main consciousness veins are the same in tantric and somatic physiology. The fifth vein of transcendental consciousness is the most important. It runs through the heart center and coincides there with the central channel. This heart center is named "good mind" (*yid-bzang-ma*) after the transcendental consciousness vein (*yid-bzang-ma rnam-shes sgyu-ba'i rtsa*). In front (east) it branches off into the red vein of sense consciousness—which itself branches off as separate veins of the five senses, to the right into a yellow vein of ego or emotional consciousness, to the left into a blue vein for thought, and in the back a green vein for the store consciousness.[4]

So the three main channels and the five consciousness veins and the veins of the five senses make up the subtle physiology of the functions of mind. The yogic view is that all mental functions are in the five veins of consciousness. These circulate throughout the body but meet in the heart center. Where they meet in the heart center is a crucial space. Distrubances in this space lead to insanity. All disease, in the Tibetan view, is caused by blocked circulation in channels of vital, mental or spiritual functions, and mental disease is particulary related to blockage at the heart center.

In a realized yogi, all the airs are transformed into their inherent wisdom-air nature and are put into the central channel. But even in un-yogically adept people like ourselves, the central vein at the heart, where it coincides with the fifth transcendental consciousness vein and branches off the other consciousness veins, is the spiritual axis of sentient existence. As one doctor, Pema Dorje, said of it (in the inevitable Tibetan style of loose analogy): "It is like a tree supporting a bird. If there is no tree, where will the bird stay? He will fly away." So mind, when this space is distorted, flies off.

The Five Causes of Insanity

The most important thing the Tibetan physican must do when first confronted with a psychiatric distrubance is to determine its cause, for the cures will vary depending on the cause and on the humoral nature of the person involved.

This means that Tibetan medicine does not treat with general anti-psychotic measures. The medicines and allied treatments have to be suitable to the patient's humoral type; if they are not, they may harm him further. And they have to be prescribed according to the individual causes of disease. Poisons and air disturbances that cause insanity demand different medicines, for example. In the case of "ghosts" and invisible forces, a main cause of mental illness according to the Tibetan system, religious practices and tantric medicines have to be used in conjunction with herbal medicines and other somatic treatments.

Since Tibetan medicine recognizes symptoms, especially psychiatric ones, as the result of innumerable subtle interwoven factors of karma, it does not look for quick cures. It takes into consideration that there is a root-poison on a spiritual level and that the effect of that poison might become worse if the symptom is forcibly displaced.

According to Burang, the general and basic cause of mental illness is thought to lie in leading a life that runs counter to one's deepest spiritual inclinations and insights and one's inherent disposition.

The initial psychiatric examination-interview will give the doctor the basic diagnostic information he needs. The process followed is similar to the one described for general medicine. First he will determine if it is a hot or cold psychiatric disease and then which humor is prevalent, if it is caused by toxins or if there is a demon involved. Even though the patient's mental state is confused or altered in some serious way, the doctor still asks questions about emotional and environmental factors in the patient's life and can tell a lot from the way the patient is "acting out." That is the interrogation part.

The parts of feeling and seeing are the same as described before, especially relying on pulse and urine analysis. In this way he determines the cause. A purely karmic case of insanity will not show up as an organic disturbance and cannot be cured by medical means. Humoral dysfunctions as primary or secondary causes, and the former is often the case in conjunction with the presence of a "ghost," are noted. Special diagnostic measures exist for determining if a "ghost" is present; these are discussed in the next chapter.

According to both Abhidharma and medical tradition there are five causes of insanity. These are: karma; grief-worry; humoral (organic) imbalance; poison (organic); and "evil spirits." These causes may work alone or in conjunction with one another.

1) Karma: In a sense, karma is responsible for all diseases, but this is not the sense in which "karmic" disease is meant. Karmic mental disease implies a specific link with destiny, a ripening of the seeds sown by former actions. For such karmic diseases there is no medicine except Dharma; nothing else is effective in counteracting negative karma. This is true for somatic as well as psychiatric disorders.

All mental sickness has its seed, it is said, in the karma of having brought suffering to someone in a past life; results are definite and even more specific. For example, if one has disturbed a person's meditation, or even just disturbed good people in general, then the effect in this life may be great sadness and depression that comes on abruptly and without any apparent cause. Similarly, if one had a predominantly malicious mind in the past, the result in this life is always to be fearful without reason.

Especially in karmic psychiatric diseases it is only the highly realized lama-doctors who can, by their special insight, determine the past actions which have created present mental disturbances.

2) Grief-Worry, etc.: In general, the psychological factors that cause insanity and mental disturbances are enumerated in relationship to the humoral causes of mental illness. This is because they create humoral disturbances as part of the symptoms of the mental illness. Many psychological functions are also associated with specific humoral divisions. For example, the "achieving bile" has its seat at the heart and is said to make a person's mind courageous or not courageous depending on how the humor is working.[5] Similarly, psychological states affect the functioning of the humors.

Psychological conditions can also work alone to produce insanity. In that case the psychological factor disturbs the life-wind (*srog-rlung*), that particular wind which is directly related to mind and which is always involved in psychiatric ailments. Obsessive and continuous mulling over of the causes of one's emotional pain, a sad love affair or loss of position, for example, are understood to produce a clinically disturbed consciousness, neurosis and psychosis.

In fact, the three basic categories of mental illness defined by the Tibetans are expressed in terms of their psychological characteristics. These are 1) fear and paranoia, 2) aggression, and 3) depression and withdrawal.

What is perhaps the most fundament and crucial psychological factor involved with the varieties of insanity is the recognition of impermanence, the very same thing which is fundamental for pursuing the Buddhist path of enlightenment. Realization of the inevitable facts of decay and death, of impermanence in all aspects of life—relationships, interests, stature, possessions—can be devastating. Especially if it is resisted, denied and repressed, then this produces a psychological tension and schizophrenic tendency.

The recognition of the essential emptiness of our egos and actions is painful and terrifying. Without the support of Dharma (in the widest sense of existing with and working with this recognition of emptiness), a tremendous panic results and leads to a repression that is elaborated in terms of ego and unconscious tendencies. This can eventually lead to psychosis.

Herein lies the crucial point. The psychological basis of insanity is the same basis for enlightenment. It all depends on whether or not it is accepted and comprehended and ultimately worked with as the key to liberation. If it is not, it becomes, because the realization is still there subconsciously, the cause of denial, repression and, ultimately, mental illness.[6]

A combination of somatic medicines, herbal mixtures, moxibustion, etc., and the practice of Dharma is used to combat mental illness produced by psychological factors. A neurotic person can practice Dharma by himself, do meditation, deepen understanding, strengthen character and steady the mind. More extreme cases, psychotics for example, cannot do these practices for themselves so a lama or other religious person must perform religious practices for them.

3) Physical (humoral) imbalances: When the humors function normally, that is when they go on their own path, then they support the health of mind and body. When they function incorrectly, they cause disease.

Excess of the psychological and emotional qualities associated with each humor aggravates the mental condition. Emotional imbalance produces humoral imbalance that is manifested as a psychiatric disturbance. All the different aspects of humoral disease theory—cause, diagnosis and cure—come into play here.

A. Air. Mental and emotional strain causes the winds or airs to increase. Thinking and concentrating on something too much, worrying about unfinished projects and unattained goals, grieving over family troubles, and becoming upset over lost articles—all these are said to disturb the wind and thus the mind, since mind and wind are bound together. Generally, it is said diseases of wind stem from overengaging in desire, lust and attachment.

Besides excitability and sadness, other symptoms of psychiatric air disorders are that a person will speak whatever comes to mind, won't remember what is said and will be unable to concentrate on or finish anything. He may cry all the time and become abruptly angry without reason. He is restless, anxious and tense.

These psychological factors lead to behavior errors which further aggravate the disturbed mental condition. For example, the psychological pain such a person experiences causes him to lose the two supports of health: diet and behavior. In this way his condition is further aggravated. Because of grief a person doesn't want to eat: fasting increases wind. He cannot sleep, which further increases the wind disorder (insomnia is a wind disease).

Psychiatric treatment first restores proper food and behavior. This is a form of naturopathy, a program of mild treatment. According to tradition, the person with a psychological air disorder

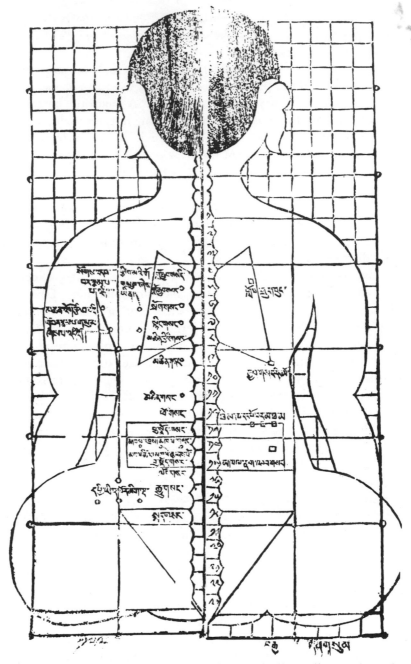

Figure 23 Second half of the medical chart showing the "secret" points located on the back and spine (see figure 22). The vertebrae are numbered in Tibetan writing starting from the base of the neck. The ones most often used in psychiatric treatment are the first, sixth and seventh. The sixth vertebra is especially important and is here called the "secret point of the life-force."

should have greasy foods, etc. which reduce air to a proper level. The patient should stay in a warm, cosy dark room. A bright room would reflect light and bright colors—thus stimulating the winds. The patient should be in an agreeable place, "a nice room with lots of flowers." The best therapeutic environment is said to be a place of great natural beauty.

In many cases, the person is advised to have sex. One symptom of psychiatric air diseases is that the sufferer often "wants to be naked and tries to take off his clothes." He is constantly thinking and talking about sex. This is all due to the desire element and its direct relation to wind. Sexual relations may help a person by satisfying desire and are therefore prescribed along with medicines.[7]

However, in some psychiatric air diseases, those caused by "ghosts" for example, sexual activity will not be therapeutic. Different medicines and treatments are applied in those cases.

Crucial to treatment of psychiatric disturbances caused by malfunctioning winds is "affectionate care." It is said that the patient should be surrounded by loving friends and family. Everyone should speak "very sweet words" of affection and concern to the patient—including and especially the doctor. The patient should be allowed to have all the things he likes best—music, books, etc. He should be kept amused and should be given everything pleasant. All of these are an ancient form of what we today call milieu and activities therapy.

If all this mild treatment of positive input from food, environment and people does not cure the patient, it will at least build his strength and resistance. It may help him enough so that he will have an occasional lucid moment, and during those periods the lama-psychiatrist can influence his consciousness by talking to him—a sort of psychotherapy.

Another somewhat mild treatment is deep or "pot" breathing exercises. Since psychiatric air diseases are often caused by malfunctions of the winds, especially "upward moving wind" and the "life supporting wind," these breathing exercises stabilize and regulate breathing and have a calming effect on the mind. They also increase and revitalize the subtle life-force, which lends a sort of existential confidence to a person, engendering a sense of well-being. This deep breathing is thought to be excellent therapy in depressive cases. It must be done correctly, however, since wrong breathing, especially holding the breath without the proper yogic wisdom, will naturally disturb the airs.

In some rare cases, yogis become insane because they have mis-manipulated the breath. This is, they fail in their attempt to put all the winds together into the central column and to transmute them into the nature of the inherent "yeshe lung"—wisdom air. Instead, they insert the impure winds into the central column where the five consciousness veins meet and this produces mental trouble, as already described.

More radical methods of psychiatric treatment include moxibustion and acupuncture. The points for these are: the top of the skull, the base of the neck—called the first vertebra in the Tibetan system (seventh cervical), the sixth vertebra (fourth thoracic), and the xiphisternal notch.[8] The last three are usually done in conjunction with each other. They are sometimes referred to as "the places of the secret vital airs." The top of the skull is the point most often used for all psychiatric disturbances.

The Tibetan medicinal massage called "kunyi" (Tib. *bsku-mnye*), literally ointment rub, is employed in psychiatric air disturbances. Herbal medicinal butter is used as the massage lubricant. It is supposed to clear the path of mind which is either blocked or polluted at the pores of the skin.

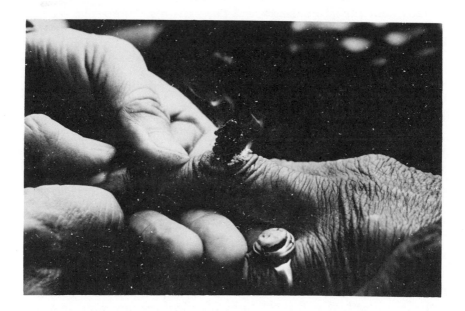

Figure 24 Moxibustion on a finger joint; here, the burning of a special herb directly on the skin. A different type of moxibustion is used for mental and emotional disorders. In it, acupuncture-like needles (of gold, silver or other metals) are inserted at specific points and heated with a substance on top of the needle.

For psychiatric wind disorders or "sok-lung," medicine butter or just butter by itself is rubbed onto the four moxa points noted above. In general, massage with medicine butter or even unmedicated oils is said to be extremely helpful in cases of heavy mental strain, worry, nervous tension, and also for old people in weak health.

One of the most popular and generally effective medicines for psychiatric air diseases are the wide range of herbal incenses which the Tibetans have developed; there are also, of course, numerous herbal medicines taken orally.

B. Bile. Psychiatric disturbances caused by bile render a person mad in a violent and rough manner, the humor bile being an outcome of aversion-anger on the mental plane. Anger and hatred, therefore, promote the overproduction of bile.

When the biles go off course in combination with emotional and psychological factors leading to the loss of the two supports of food and behavior, then the madness that results is classified as being of a bile nature, although it also involves a disturbance of air.

A violent psychosis results. The patient speaks harshly and abusively to others, disturbs and breaks things, and may injure or even kill other beings. He is constantly angry, dwells on past annoyances and is high strung. It is thought that such a person may have to be restrained and given rough treatment and punishment.

Behaviorally, the patient should stay quietly in a cool place like a breezy garden or near a river bed or a mountain stream. The colors and environment surrounding him should have a cooling effect.

His food and beverage should also be of a cool nature. Coffee, alcohol, stimulants, fatty foods, and eggs should be avoided. Special medicinal baths are prescribed for clearing the air channel of mental function which is blocked due to excess bile (for details, see note H of Chapter 78, page 189).

C. Phlegm. Confusion, ignorance and sloth promote the production of phlegm. The person who becomes mad because of excess of the humor phlegm displays a pathologically phlegmatic nature. He becomes completely withdrawn, silent, inactive and sullen.

Such a person refuses to eat and tends to roll his eyes upwards and to have dizzy spells. He puts things in places and then can't remember where. In addition to being silent, he is especially closed-minded.

Highly affectionate treatment is applied to draw him out. He is induced into activity whenever possible. He must have plenty of exercise. Massage is also helpful here because it imparts physical movement to the body, even if passive, and produces warmth (phlegm is cold). The patient must stay in a warm bright place where friends and family are with him telling him stories and "sweet words." His food and beverages must be those to combat phlegm.

Besides these mild treatments, herbal medicines must be administered. Also, forced vomiting with medicine butter will be used to clear the channel of wind and mind blocked by phlegm. Sometimes a hot medicine bath will be helpful for this same purpose, or an application (fomentation) of the medicine butter or even the herbal bath mixture.

The modes of madness associated with the three humoral types can be said to correspond generally with modern classifications of known psychiatric disturbances. For example, madness caused by phlegm corresponds to catatonia, or what the *Diagnostic and Statistical Manual of Mental Disorders* (which contains concise definitions of the categories of mental illness according to modern medical theory) calls "schizophrenia, catatonic type, withdrawn" (by number 295:24), "general inhibition manifested by stupor, mutism, negativism or waxy flexibility. In time, some cases deteriorate to a vegetative state."[9]

Similarly, the violent bile type of madness can be said to be like (295:23), "schizophrenia, catatonic type, excited," "marked by excessive and sometimes violent motor activity and excitement." The wind type of madness corresponds to classical schizophrenia (295), "characteristic disturbances of thinking, mood, and behavior."[10]

4) *Poison*: Toxins are held to be a direct cause of insanity. In such cases the mind becomes completely confused, strength wanes and the radiance of good health disappears, especially in the face. The weakness of body caused by poison does not get better with the intake of good food and essences because the poison has not been cleared away. The mental confusion of psychiatric disturbances caused by poison is called "deep illusion." The victim doesn't know at all where his mind is going or he may alternate between normal lucidity and completely illusionary thinking and unawareness.

Poison may be a specific toxin or may be the poisonous combination of otherwise non-toxic foods and beverages or may be the slow, gradual build-up of toxic substances in the body. Herbal and animal medicines are used to treat the insanity caused by poison.

Again, modern psychiatry also classifies mental diseases in relationship to nutritional disorders and to poison.

5) *Demons or Evil Spirits*: A "demon" or "evil spirit" which causes insanity is a demonic effect that overcomes a person and then takes over his actions of body, speech and mind. This negative energy penetrates the conscious psyche of an individual because the person is psychologically weak and has no resistance. The "ghost" or "demon" may be the sole cause of the insanity or may be present along with psychological, humoral or poisonous causes.

The symptoms of the presence of a "ghost" in psychiatric disturbances are that the person is abruptly changed in his behavior and acts very differently than before. How he acts depends on the kind of "ghost" he is affected by. The classifications of various ghosts are, then, classifications of different kinds of psychoses. This Tibetan system shows a very ancient and detailed system of the classification of insanity based upon psychological, behavioral, and physical symptoms that are understood as being of the effects of "ghosts."

Treatment is elaborate because it entails many special tantric anti-"ghost" procedures and of course the employment of religious medicine, since being overcome by "demons" and negative forces is specifically karmic even though it may or may not have psychological or organic contributing causes. Different and complicated herbal treatments exist for insanity caused by different "ghosts."

Some of these psychiatric treatments are those which we have not mentioned previously in relation to general medicine. These are very occult procedures for countering the evil effect of "ghosts" by using other things which have also been tainted by evil. Included among such things are the blood of murdered people. Tibetan doctors usually carry a supply of dried blood from a murdered person for these purposes. In addition, amulets etc. are used to ward off these negative forces in the first place.

Mantras are also employed as therapy, and extensive religious practices often have to be done for the patient who is too incapacitated to do them for himself. In general, mantras and medicines compounded from herbal and animal extracts are used to cure psychiatric disturbances caused by harmful spirits.

Because demons are a basic vehicle by which insanity is understood in the Tibetan system, "psychiatry" is synonymous with diseases caused by invisible spirits, and since the three psychiatric chapters included here in translation from the *Gyu-zhi* are about "demons," it seems best to go into some detail about them.

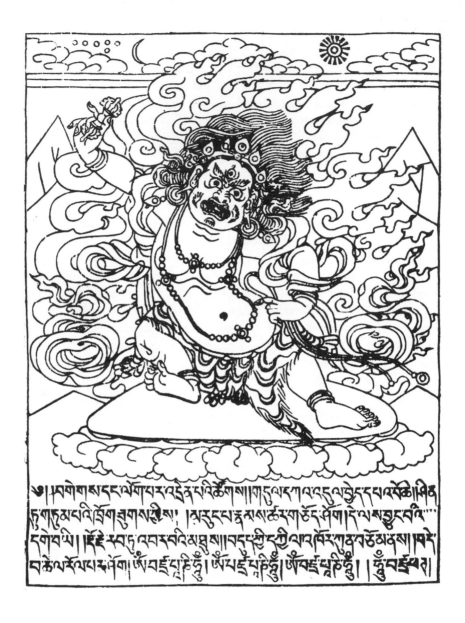

Figure 25 Vajrapani, Chanadorje, the wrathful embodiment and power aspect of enlightenment. He vowed to protect whomever invokes the name of the Medicine Buddha. Ritual practice of Vajrapani is used against all demonic influences and elemental spirits, especially those who cause disorders of the central nervous system (as described in Chapter 80 of the *Gyu-zhi's* Third Tantra). The prayer to him inscribed here ends with the mantra HUNG VAJRA PHAT, a mantra also used to treat strokes, epilepsy, etc.

9

"Demons" in Medical Psychiatry

The Third Tantra of the *Gyu-zhi* contains five chapters specifically on diseases caused by spirits, and three of these are about the demons (*gdon*) who cause mental illness. Scattered throughout the *Gyu-zhi's* one hundred and fifty-six chapters, however, is much material pertaining to mental illness. Chapter headings don't always reflect the broad range of material which they contain, but the ones with which we are dealing here are exclusively about mental illness and the evil spirits that are thought to cause it.

These five chapters on diseases caused by spirits are classified together as one etiological group and are sometimes referred to as the *Gyu-zhi's* section on psychiatry, psychiatry being synonomous, in the classical Ayurvedic sense, with ailments caused by unseen forces. The chapters are as follows:

Chapter 77: Elemental spirits (*'Byung-po'i gdon*). These invade the psyche, are of 18 kinds, and have specific traits.

Chapter 78: Madness demons (*sMyo-byed-kyi gdon*). These invade the psyche alone or in conjunction with aberrations of poison, humors and emotions.

Chapter 79: Amnesia demons (*brJed-byed-kyi gdon*). These are literally the "demons who bring forgetfulness."

Chapter 80: Demonic rulers of planets (*gZaa-yi gdon*). They cause epilepsy.

Chapter 81: Serpent-spirit demons (*kLu'i gdon*). These cause leprosy.

All of the "demons" listed above as specific causes of different psychiatric disorders are called by the Tibetan word *gdon,* 'don.' *gDon* is commonly translated as "ghost," "evil spirit," or "demon." But to most modern Westerners "ghosts" are the fabrications of a childish mind, imaginary spectral creatures who haunt houses and the like. The word "demon," similarly, conjures up images of diabolical fiends, mythological creatures, nothing real. And similarly again for evil spirits, external negative forces, and so on.

We can't imagine how any sophisticated religion, philosophy or culture—not to mention medicine—could put any credence in what we assume to be the mere figments of imagination. So how is it that Tibetan Buddhist medical psychiatry places these "demons" at the center of their system?

What are these "Demons"?

To the Tibetans, "demon" is a symbolic term. It represents a wide range of forces and emotions which are normally beyond conscious control and all of which prevent well-being and spiritual development.

To gain some idea of the extent of forces covered by the term, one has only to consider the famous "four devils" who appear throughout Buddhist literature and who represent obstacles on the path of awakening. They are: the devil of the aggregates—frailty of body and mind; the devil of the kleshas—the devastating power of afflictive emotions; the devil of pleasure—the alluring trap of comfort; and the devil of death—who surely comes and cuts this life and with it the opportunity for spiritual growth.

Obviously, none of these is a devil in the narrow sense of the word. These "devils," like other "demons," are outer and inner factors that exert their influence subconsciously or almost irresistably, obstructing the realization of higher aspirations.

These forces range from subtle, inherited and unconscious tendencies to overwhelming drives like sex, and for the practitioner, according to Patrul Rinpoche, they can include such "demons" as laziness, lust, bad companions, dualistic thinking, hypersensitivity, increased emotionality, attachment to wealth, sectarianism, spiritual pride, and clinging to tranquility.[11]

The lamas often compare the rise of such negative forces against the practitioner who is trying to refine his ordinary consciousness to the situation in a country where the people want positive change and the ruling powers do all they can to prevent it. Clearly, then, in a psychoanalytic sense, these demons are in the role of the id trying to obstruct the super-ego's higher promptings.

Thus, demons are primarily a psychological phenomenon associated with the multitude of mental and emotional obscurations. Among all kinds of demons, there are mainly said to be two: those born of hope and those born of doubt. And these, in turn, arise from the basic ignorance which grasps at the illusion of a permanent "self." This ego-grasping, which Shantideva calls "that great ghost," is said to cause all injury, fear and pain in the world. This is a central theme of Buddhism.

As Ma-Chig-La, a marvelous 12th century yogini, explained to her disciple:

> What we call a Demon is very, very huge, and colored all black. Whoever sees one is truly terrified and trembles from head to foot—but Demons don't really exist!

> The truth of the matter is this: Anything whatsoever that obstructs the attainment of liberation is a Demon. Even loving and affectionate relatives can become Demons if they hinder your practice. But the greatest Demon of them all is belief in a self as an independent and lasting principle. If you don't destroy this clinging to a self, Demons will just keep lifting you up and letting you down. [12]

However, even though they are understood to be psychological in this way, some types of "demons" are thought to have an outer existence. But while the common Tibetan may vividly believe in these external negative forces as actual "demons," learned Tibetans, as Theodore Burang explained, regard them "as mental entities or projections (mostly of a lower order) or as psychic fields of force, either natural or contrived." [13]

It seems important to remember in this regard that before the advent of Buddhism, Tibet was a thoroughly shamanistic civilization given to the belief in all kinds of personified forces of mind and nature as devils and deities and the like. This cultural tendency to see things in such terms was incorporated into Buddhism, its meaning transformed.

Furthermore, Buddhism itself posits the existence of all kinds of sentient creatures in the wheel of life, some of whom have no physical bodies. Hell, for example, is said to be a projected state of mind experienced with a subtle or light body and arrived at by the force of one's own interminable vicious actions. Heaven, similarly, is divinely pleasurable and experienced with the mental light body or even no body at all, just mind—the highest heavenly states are contemplative absorptions.

Moreover, in the realm of the hungry ghosts, there are two classes of spirits: the actual hungry ghosts, who harm no one but suffer by themselves, and the other tortured spirits, mind-streams that roam the universe in states of agitation and unhappiness, inflicting harm almost helplessly, habitually. These latter group are what are usually indicated by the term "outer demons."

And even these so-called outer demons have a relationship to the psyche; they are part of an interplay between the microcosm and the macrocosm, and in this relationship mind is chief. For example, some types of demons are associated with the elements of nature. They are called forth, as it were, by a disturbance of the inner elements in the body—and this may be true of the "elemental spirits" who cause schizophrenia. Negative emotions disturb the inner elements, the inner elements disturb the outer elements, and attacks by the spirits of the elements result; these are expressed as the demons of wind, hail, etc. Thus, natural disasters are said to arise in response to the collective emotional disturbances of human beings.

The Tibetans are perfectly comfortable classifying this wide range of forces under the one heading of "demon," although the modern Western mind doubtless finds it hard to grasp. Nevertheless, even in our own language that which we call a "demon" can mean (according to Webster) "an undesirable or evil emotion, trait or state personified," while a "devil" can be "a mood, passion, or quality that possesses, incites or disturbs."

Thus, in the pre-Freudian terms of Tibet, "demons" and "devils" are appropriate names for the forces of life and emotion that can drive the mind insane.

In order to get a still better sense of exactly what the Tibetans mean by "demon," *gdon,* we may profitably look at the word more closely.

gDon is the same Tibetan word as the future tense for the verb *'don,* which means "to cause to come out or come forth, to drive forth." That is the original meaning of the verb; with changes of usage it came to mean more "to take out" than "to give out." It is also used in conjunction with the word "mantra" and means "to pronounce a magic formula" (*sngags- 'don-pa*), which we know means to emit a primordial vibration in order to effect a change on a subtle level of consciousness and existence.[14]

So, the more proper sense of the noun *gdon* is as a "radiating effect." In the case of "ghosts," "demons," and "evil spirits," they are understood to be those beings or forces that radiate negative effects.

We have to return to basic Buddhist philosophy to understand this further. The whole world is, in the Buddhist view, impermanent, a dynamic manifestation of vibrations. We are a "bundle of perceptions," as it were. Nothing is solid, neither our bodies, nor our egos, nor the mountains, nor the stars. Everything is a temporary and changing configuration of minute particles of existence which we call atoms and the Buddhist call dharmas—without a capital "D." And even these particles themselves are vibrations, not solid in essence but changing. This universe is like an immense field of electromagnetic energy.

Therefore, the whole of conditioned existence consists of radiations of energy vibrations emitted as rays or as fields of force and at varying rates of speed and thus solidity, intersecting and interacting in accordance with the harmonics of karmic balance.

And since mental obscurations are at the root of these manifestations and since all beings in this world have a transitory existence appropriate to their karma, that is, appropriate to the vibrational course they have set for themselves through the acts of body, speech and mind in countless lives, the realms of conditioned existence are populated with many kinds of creatures, entities and forces, not all of whom are immediately visible and some of whom are without embodied forms.

The *gdon,* according to this outer interpretation, are "beings" or forces whose existence is a coagulation as a direct result of bad and particularly poisonous karmic vibrations.

Since almost everything in Buddhism has at least three levels of interpretation, we can approach these "demons" on the psychological or inner level. Just as, for example, all the realms of samsara exist externally, they also exist internally. We are constantly dying and being reborn from moment to moment as gods, animals, ghosts, denizens of hells, and on and on wherever our thoughts, emotions and actions take us.

The psychological interpretation of the so-called "demons" and "ghosts" is that on some levels they are the embodied forms we give to our negative projections, those dark forces in ourselves which are too awful to admit into consciouness and which are then projected outward and turned against ourselves. In terms of Western psychology, these could be explained as ego-alien unconscious material and impulses that are projected as destructive forces that are perceived as an outer form which then possess us (audio-visual hallucinations etc.). Those are our own ghosts, so to speak. That is projection in one life.

Ghosts are also the imprints of mental habits and thought patterns whose unconscious hold is so strong that they are constantly projected, unawares, onto the world. This produces distortions in the perception of reality as well as all kinds of inappropriate or "insane" behavior.

For the inner point of view, these "demons" can also be explained as the negative archetypes of the collective unconscious, archetypes which overtake us from within. Jung maintained that evil comes from the collective unconscious and it is this unconscious which "possesses" us. "The tremendous power of the 'objective psychic'", wrote Jung, "has been named 'demon' or 'God' in all epochs with the sole exception of the recent present. We have become so bashful in matters of religion that we correctly say 'unconscious'...."[15]

From the absolute or "secret" point of view, the true nature of these "demons" is voidness. They have no self-nature and are non-existent as such. This is illustrated in one part of the life story of Milarepa, Tibet's famous poet, yogi and saint.

One day Milarepa left his meditation cave to get some wood. On returning, he found several demons sitting in his cave and taunting him. Milarepa tried everything he could think of to subdue and overcome them. First he tried to propitiate them as the local deities of the place, then he used the meditation and mantra of a wrathful Buddha, but they continued to attack him. Then suddenly, in realization, he said, "Through the mercy of Marpa [his guru], I have already fully realized that all beings and all phenomena are one's own mind. The mind itself is a transparency of Voidness."[16] With that, the demons vanished.

Commenting on this famous story, Trungpa Rinpoche explained, "This was the beginning of Milarepa's period of learning how to subjugate the demons, which is the same thing as transmuting the emotions. It is with our emotions that we create demons and gods. Those things we want out of our lives and the world are the demons;

those things which we would draw to us are the gods and goddesses."[17]

Since the source of the demons is mind, the basic premise of Tibetan Buddhist psychology is that if we can control the mind and the wild negative emotions, we can protect ourselves against these spectral negative influences and be rid of them.

Regardless of how the demons are interpreted, their particular effects are the varieties of psychopathology, and these can only arise in us when the mind is unstable and inflamed with emotions to such an extent that the personality is no longer functionally integrated. Burang has explained this in terms of the five skandhas, the psycho-physical energies that compose the personality and mental existence. When the five skandhas are discordant, then, he says, "a displacement of the layers of personality" ensues and "the result is a kind of split in consciousness which the Western psychiatrist encounters in schizophrenia."

Such displacements are a form of mental illness that may be treated on their own (with a kind of emotional or mental shock therapy), but it is this condition of displaced aggregates or skandhas that is "conducive to the occupation of the component parts of the personality by vehicles from the outside."[18]

While demonic forces arise, in general, from the negative states of mind, different kinds of them have specific causes ascribed to them.

In the Tibetan tradition, some "ghosts" and "evil spirits" are said to be created at the time of death; these are "ghosts" in the Western sense of the term, spirits of the dead. Tibetan Buddhism holds that the consciousness that leaves a dying person is most greatly affected by the state of mind at the time of death. If a person panics for some reason or other or is full of hatred, fear or strong attachment, the panic or hatred energy projection becomes very solid, i.e., a "ghost."

If the dying person is extraordinarily attached to his wealth, for example, and all his thoughts cling to it at death, then instead of his consciousness going into the intermediate regions before rebirth, part of it is drawn to the object of attachment and it hovers around the thing collecting into an astral "ghost" form interfering with, for example, the people who subsequently receive the money.

Suicides and murders are also thought to be very inauspicious modes of dying because such strong negative clingings and panic are involved. That sort of negative energy is usually bound to form some sort of ghost at death.[19] In cases of murder, suicide and sudden death when there has been no preparation of the dying consciousness with the usual means of prayer etc., a lama is most always called in to perform an exorcism to prevent the formation of a ghost—or to get rid of it. This kind of ghost is said to have a life-span limited to nine years; after that it dissolves.

Still other kinds of demons and negative entities are those created purposefully by the negative projections of a sorcerer. A person with advanced psychic powers, a black magician you could say, who understands and can manipulate the cosmic forces in himself and the universe can create forces specifically to harm other beings and drive them insane; these are the "evil curse ghosts" of Chapter 77. Unlike a spiritually realized being, the person who projects such forces has a strong ego and selfish passions. He uses his powers for his own evil goals.

In Buddhism, of course, psychic powers are never to be sought for their own sake. They develop by themselves while one is treading the path to enlightenment and they are to be used as instruments of wisdom and compassion. This kind of possible abuse is one reason why the psycho-physical keys to tantric processes and psychic forces, in religion and medicine, are carefully guarded by the lamas and holders of the lineage.

Classifications of Spirits Causing Mental Illness

Besides the listing from the *Gyu-zhi,* there are numerous systems of classification of demons and spirits within the Tibetan tradition and Buddhism in general. Here we are only discussing those which cause mental illness. But whether we are discussing the tantric, medical or general Buddhist approach, we find that all agree on this: evil spirits, ghosts, demons and negative forces are the result of obscurations of mind.

In other words, their origin is the three poisons, mental states which arise with ego. The three poisons generate three basic classes of *gdon,* demons, or malignant effects.

These *gdon* come under the wider heading of the term "gek" (*bgegs*), which literally means a hindrance or obstruction. Among the 84,000 "geks" referred to in the Sutras, a number that accords with the 84,000 mental defilements enumerated by the Buddha and the 84,000 diseases arising from them, there are 1,080 spirits who are referred to as the sentient "demons" and malignant spirits we know as *gDon*. These 1,080 "geks" are described as causing faults of mind. It is sometimes said that 360 of them arise from the mental poison of ignorance, 360 from the mental poison of desire and 360 from the mental poison of hatred.[20]

While there are many different systems for classifying "demons" and negative forces, *gdon* are generally put into three groups: 1) demonic spirits from above; 2) demonic spirits from below; and 3) demonic spirits from in between.

The demonic spirits from above are the "rulers of planetary forces" (Tib. *gzaa-yi gdon*). They are not the planets as phenomena themselves but are their negative demonic effects. They are subdivided into five categories corresponding to the five elements. These planetary forces are the "demons" described in Chapter 80 of the Third Tantra of the *Gyu-zhi*. Their poisonous effect is that of causing epilepsy, sudden paralysis and strokes.

They are said mainly to attack the brain and the nervous system and to strike very suddenly: sudden unconsciousness is one of the symptoms.

These planetary forces are like the other *gdon*. They embody a poison (obscuration) and in that existence travel through time and space radiating poisonous effects. If you cross their paths, you are struck very suddenly with their effect, which is epilepsy, twitches, paralysis and seizures (an appropriate word). Coming into face-to-face confrontation with them, you are immediately knocked out.[21]

In general, it is said to be difficult to treat diseases caused by demonic planetary influences with regular medicine. Treatment through mantra, meditation and rituals is recommended. One tantric medicine used for these diseases is the fresh blood of a murdered person on the tip of a knife. If it is immediately touched to the lip of the patient, he will recover (dried blood will do if necessary).

Because of their relation to planets, certain days of the lunar month have been specified by Tibetan psychiatry on which these demonic forces strike in a rhythmical frequency of astrological significance.[22]

The "demonic spirits from below" are the negative effects of the serpent-spirits or *nagas* (Tib. *klu'i gdon*). The nagas live primarily in the ocean. Their demonic effect (described in Chapter 81 of the Third Tantra of the *Gyu-zhi*) is the cause of leprosy, as well as a host of other diseases and disturbances.

While it is not too surprising to us to find epileptic disorders categorized as psychiatric disturbances, since they have sometimes been viewed that way in the West, the inclusion of leprosy in the same etiological group with psychiatric disease seems extremely strange.

In Tibetan view, however, skin diseases are thought to be closely related to psychological phenomena since the inner airs related to mind interface with the outer air and outer world through the medium of the skin. But leprosy in particular is considered as practically the primal psychiatric disease, the result of the irreparable bad karma of humanity. The idea is that by dint of humanity's grotesque and cruel thoughts, words and actions such negativity was generated that a disharmony of the humors arose as a general condition. The serpent-spirits, nagas, could then easily exert their poisonous effects on people, and the horrible disease of leprosy manifested. The 81st chapter, which discusses these nagas, leprosy and the progressive degeneration of the human race, is supposed to be the most esoteric section of the *Gyu-zhi.*

Some stories in Tibetan mythology support the view that the nagas are the primal source of bad spirits and that all demonic spirits causing serious mental illness originate from them (this parallels the idea that they arise from ignorance rather than desire or hatred). One Tibetan myth tells how even Vajrapani, emanation of Buddha power, was once unable to subdue the naga king Vashudhari. Vashudhari just breathed his steamy vapor on Vajrapani and Vajrapani turned black and powerless. It took the fabulous divine bird, Garuda, to subdue the naga king.[23]

More than anything else this story points out that the powerful force of evil karma is not easily restrained. Leprosy is the most gruesome symbolic mirror of psychological filth and sickness; we think we can hide from our spiritual deformity, since it is not immediately visible, but we can't. It eats away at us and creates mental and physical disease.

This is a little paradigm that reveals the basic psychosomatic disease theory of Tibetan medicine. But unlike modern psychosomatic disease theory, which only involves one individual in one lifetime, the Tibetan view is built on the premise of individual "psycho-moral continuum" or karma of past lives, and moreover, on the interconnectedness of everything and everybody in this life and previously for uncountable eons, so that the cumulative collective karmic force expresses itself in time-periods, often as specific diseases. The modern scourge of cancer, for example, could be explained in this way.

Demons from "in between" cause a range of mental illness from slight depression to complete insanity. This whole class of demons from "in between" is said to attack the heart center (where the function of mind resides) and therefore to engender loss of control of mind. These demonic forces are said to enter the body through the psychic channel in the ring finger, a channel leading to the heart center.[24]

The demons from "in between" are sub-divided into four families: royal, aristocratic, common and "butcher" class, i.e. very aggressive. Mental diseases caused by the royal family of "in between" demons are the easiest to treat. The aggressive "butcher" class is hardest to treat, and the healer of the patient affected by them is said to be subject to their strong negative influence. He is therefore advised to use lots of protection when treating such patients.

Further, the "in between" demons are of three different types—male, female, and neuter. These types correspond to the three main mental poisons which produce them—anger, attachment, and ignorance, respectively—and their effects vary accordingly.

The practice of various somatic medical therapies can help the mental diseases caused by these types of demons, but most effective is said to be mantra and meditation and the taking of special "mantra pills," a tantric medicine made by lamas and empowered with the force and blessings of hundreds of thousands of mantras and also actual written mantras which are rolled into "pills."

The Tibetan doctor or lama-doctor must know demonology in order to perform his duties as a psychiatrist (there is no separate class of psychiatrists). Knowing the conspicuous traits of the various demons, he can recognize their presence through the patient's behavior which reflects the demon's character. There is also an astrological aspect involved in recognizing one demon from another, since some are stronger during particular time cycles.

Besides observing a psychiatric patient's behavior and case history, a doctor may diagnose the presence of a ghost through pulse and urine analysis.

Additionally, the presence of a demon may be diagnosed by certain marks on the body. In his commentary on the *Gyu-zhi*, Mipham Rinpoche enumerates the following physical signs of the different families of spirits from "in between" (and adds a fifth family to the above listing). If the brightness of the eyes has deteriorated, if there are changes in the blood vessels in the whites of the eyes, if there are very small black dots on the whites of the eyes, or if the eyes look blurred or scratched, these are all signs of possession by a kingly or royal spirit (*rgyal-po*). Mipham Rinpoche notes that this group is the one most often responsible for causing madness.

Signs of the other classes of spirits are: fleshy bumps on the right elbow in the shape of the Tibetan letter "ra" (aristocratic); flesh on the left elbow in the shape of a spear (priestly); on the left knee in the form of the letter "ga" without its horizontal stroke (common); and on the soles of the feet in the shape of a fish or the letter "nya" (lowest or butcher).[25]

There is a type of pulse that indicates the presence of a ghost; it is called "ghost-pulse" (*gdon-rtsa*). This pulse is characterized by highly irregular or patternless beating. For example, it may beat 1, 2, 3, stop then 1, 2, 3, 4, 5, stop, then double beat. This pulse is described in the first chapter of the Fourth Tantra.

The divinatory process in urine analysis is considerably more elaborate. It involves the use of an astrological diagram (very likely of Chinese origin) which is placed over a bowl of urine to form nine squares. It is called "mebaga" (*sme-ba-dga*). Its nine squares represent the residence of a group of nine spirits called "sadak" (*sa-bdag*) or ground-owner demons.

The nine divisions of "sadak" are assigned to the nine squares as indicated in figure 26.

There is a special kind of urine bubble that looks exactly like a fish-eye (and is known by that name); it is the one that indicates the presence of a ghost. When it arises in the urine and goes into one of the nine squares, then the doctor knows which kind of ghost is harming the person.

These nine ground-owner demons are not, as a named group, mentioned in the psychiatric texts of the *Gyu-zhi*. This is because the

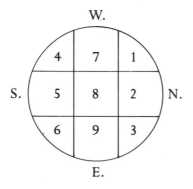

1. gods (*lHa*)
2. men (*mi*)
3. ghosts (*gDon*)
4. cremation ground (*dur-sa*)
5. house (*khang*)
6. fields (*shing*)
7. ancestors (*pha-mes*)
8. self (*rang*)
9. progeny (*bu-tsha*)

Figure 26 The nine squares of the "sadak."

group in Chapter 77, the elementals, are partly taken directly from Indian tradition while these sadak are pre-Buddhist Bon deities of Tibet that were incorporated into Tibetan Buddhism. Even so, these elementals and sadak overlap as types—ancestor ghosts, gods-ghosts, etc. Furthermore, they share typical demonical qualities—like being associated with and jealous of specific places.

The sadak also number generally among the kinds of ghosts who cause madness. Some lamas and doctors hold that sadak in particular provide psychological disturbances to meditators who get into trouble while in deep meditation.[26]

That there are many kinds and names of "demons" gives us a sense of the breadth and variety of negative forces which the Tibetan system recognizes. The Tibetans have an elaborate view of the dark side of the mostly invisible, immaterial worlds of existence, much as they also hold an elaborate and panoramic view of limitless radiant Buddha-realms.

The Tibetan enumeration of "ghosts" and their specific qualities and behavior is an examination of the way negativity exists in the macrocosm as well as in the microcosm of an individual's psyche. "Ghosts" and "evil spirits" are not regarded simply as the projections of an unhealthy mind. For although they arose from projections, they are said to be real in the relative sense. That is, they have to be dealt with. They arise from habits and passions in the manner of all interdependent-arising as described in Buddhism.

The "demons" can thus be understood as mental habits which become stronger and stronger until they take form—like the way subject-object division of events in a day find their way into our dreams. The dreams are not true, but they feel true when we are in them. All samsara, the Tibetans say, is like this; ghosts are the same.

That the categories of demons overlap so much is indicative of the richness of the culture from which they come and the deeply ingrained place they have within it. This overlapping can be helpful to us in trying to understand what Tibetans mean by "demons" because we cannot have too rigid an idea of the shapes and forms and names of the "evil spirits," but rather we can get an impression of their types and actions.

For example, there are demons called ground-owner demons. As their name implies, they are very possessive of their place and very harmful to anyone who abuses it. But many other kinds of demons and malicious spirits have the quality of being angered when other beings invade their space. This is one way that the confrontation, intersection and "possession" occurs.

We find in Chapter 77 of the Third Tantra that one of the ways in which all the elemental spirits mentioned there invade a person's being and make him crazy in the manner of their own dispositions is that the person has defiled the ghost's place. Usually that person, it is said, also has some weakness of mind that permits him to be influenced by these negative effects.

One simple thing that this points to is that Tibetan medical psychiatry takes into account the effect of the "vibrations" of the environment on the mental state of the individual. The emanations of different places are associated with different poisonous effects. For example, the negative influences of various places in terms of the spirits who reside there were enumerated by the great fourteenth century philosopher-saint, Longchenpa. In speaking about places that are either bad or good for meditation, he says that funeral monuments and certain shrinerooms have poisonous emanations due to the male mischievous spirits (rgyal-'gong) who "make the mind feel giddy and thoughts of hatred grow." Female spirits (bsen-mo) are in places with a languorous atmosphere such as caverns where "lust is born and feelings of depression and elation grow in excess."27

The psychiatric chapters of the Gyu-zhi also say that staying alone in deserted places—or just staying alone in general—can send a person over the brink—i.e., a "ghost" gets in at that time. This shows the importance of being sensitive to emanations of the environment as well as a clear awareness of the adverse effects of isolation on human beings, humans, that is, who are not strengthened by Dharma practice, for people practicing Dharma are encouraged to stay alone. Serious yogis spend years alone in meditational retreats. Great tantrikas meditate in cremation grounds because so many powerful negative spirits are there to be transformed and bound to the Dharma; they add power to the tantrika's practice. This contrast points out how Dharma practice helps one resist the poison (madness-ghosts) and to transmute the poison into the nectar of awareness.

There is a similar contrast with the ancestral spirits who are found within various classifications. For example, among the sadaks is an ancestral demon whom we may think of as the spirit of genetic inheritance. An ancestral ghost is also listed among the elementals of Chapter 77. They differ slightly, perhaps, in how and where they rule but essentially they are the same, just as they are recognized and worshipped in many societies. One could say that this ancestral spirit represents the negative forces and mental aberration that result from cutting oneself off from one's psychic, family and cultural heritage—

the unskillful cutting off. Again, by contrast, in Dharma practice it is necessary to cut oneself off from attachments and inherited dispositions, but this is done in a skillful way.

Evil Spirits and the Medicine of Dharma Practice

Two predominate themes emerge in the Dharma view of "demons". One, from the level of absolute truth, they do not exist. Like everything else, they have no self-nature. They are in fact empty. Two, from the level of relative truth, they have conditioned existence. One should protect oneself from their negative influence.

The lamas explain that ghosts arise from conceptualization; they come from the duality of mind. Whether they are real or not real is up to the practice of the perceiver. If one has the "pure vision" of the Vajrayana wisdom mind, then they are experienced as pure phenomena, just as samsara and nirvana are inseparably experienced as the tri-kaya.

Approaching ghosts and spirits from the level of absolute truth, we realize the nature of emptiness, theirs and ours, so nothing can harm us. The wisdom of the present awareness of emptiness is the Dharmakaya; nothing can affect it. By realizing shunyata, all sickness and negativity is subdued or dissolved. Those distinctions simply do not exist.

In this wisdom there is no hope or fear. Therefore even if a "demon" appeared to rush towards one with a flaming dagger, the person whose mind is identified with emptiness is immovable, adamantine, and no demon can harm him. The demon disappears. All is the primordially pure nature of mind. Then even protective measures against negative spirits (exorcisms and the like) are subsumed in the realization of emptiness. As said in a tantra:

> When the nature of Mind has been realized
> As making offerings and performing exorcism
> And all other sorts of work and duties
> (Then you understand that) everything is encompassed by
> it.[28]

So we can defeat all demons and ghosts with the supreme medicine— the realization of radiant emptiness, absolute truth, from which compassion spontaneously arises.

On a relative level, these negative forces and demons are understood to have an actual existence, but the absolute truth, that all phenomena has no self-nature and is generated by the ego-habits of countless lives, is kept in mind. In writing about Buddhism and evil forces, H. V. Guenther said:

> Religion has symbolized the helpful forces and powers into gods and the evil ones into demons and the Devil, all of which for philosophy is but a medley of deceptive veils and misleading simplifications. Buddhism seems to be more on the philosophical side; it rejects the primitive belief in gods and demons, but as it developed it did not like the "intellectual" try to kill the primitive within us.[29]

The lamas emphasize that we should not attempt to limit the wide dimensions of existence in general and "demons" in particular to flat and linear concepts which may be easier for us to understand. They refuse to relate to demons only as psychological phenomena in the Western sense, although they are of course psychological phenomena in the Buddhist sense that whatever perceptions we harbor we eventually materialize. Attempts to limit them to psychological terms acceptable to modern psychology are, they say, typical of the materialistic habits of modern man. It is true, they say, that demons are not real and don't exist from an absolute point of view, and further that the ones in question here are expressed in symbolic terms from primitive beliefs but, they say, until we recognize emptiness these are still invisible negative energies and whether spawned from within or without their negative effects are very much to be reckoned with.

Even without having fully realized emptiness, the person who practices Dharma knows the world is a materialized projection of mind, the result of dualistic conceptions. But obscurations are still there and the person still clings to the projections, to the sense of being separate subject and the outside being separate object. So one can intellectually understand the ghosts as an aspect of mind, but the "ghosts" can still cause harm.

An illustration of this is the story of a yogi whose meditation was terribly disturbed by a snake which kept coming and distracting him with fear. His guru gave him advice on dealing with it, but to no avail. Finally the guru said to take a stick (not to bother with a knife) and mark an "X" on the snake's belly, that that would certainly defeat the snake. When the yogi did this, he found later that the cross was marked on his own belly. Then he recognized the nature of mind and was liberated.

Compassion is also understood to be a supreme medicine and protection against ghosts and demons. For according to Dharma psychology, when we try to reject something, we actually become more vulnerable to it. We come to realize this through the practice of meditation and watching the mind. We let unconscious material surface without rejecting or identifying with it. And thus it begins to lose its power over us. Seeing the nature of emptiness, even if only for a moment, compassion arises simultaneously.

In this case one does not struggle with the demons but feels glad to have the opportunity to purify one's karma and wishes that through the difficulties one is experiencing others will not have to suffer. The lamas say that such a positive and altruistic attitude is enough to make the obstacles or demons vanish by themselves.

Besides developing compassion and the recognition of emptiness (wisdom) on the absolute level, there are other relative tantric practices employed for protection against these negative forces. For example, in Vajrayana the mandala or mystic circle is used in part in this way. It protects against demons as a first step to integrating consciousness—for demons and evil forces, by definition, prevent one from realizing the higher levels of awareness.

The mandala is a cosmogram structured so that its outer portion represents an impenetrable foil to negative demonic effects. One visualizes oneself as being protected within the ordained holy structure. Or one may visualize oneself as identified with a wrathful meditational deity (yidam) and then send out from various chakras lights which turn into tantric ritual weapons which form a circle (sometimes visualized as being miles in diameter) protecting one against disruptive negative energies which might prevent one from integrating with the wisdom consciousness. This practice also involves believing that no harm can penetrate to oneself and not seeing oneself in the ordinary way but as an aspect of Buddhahood.

Practice of the ritual meditations or sadhanas of the wrathful deities such as Mahakala, Vajrakilaya, Vajrapani, Hayagriva, Garuda, Kalachakra, etc., demolishes demons. Herbert Guenther has described the psychological significance of such meditative visualizations.

> All that which is not and cannot be clearly understood as it rises out of the depth of the psychic life of man, and which

not only disturbs but also frequently dominates him, has been concretely formulated as "demons." Where these demons are not a mere figure of speech they are the vivid expression of man's active engagement in experienced reality, as it is felt in horror or ecstasy. This feeling that what we can sense points to something hidden, unfathomable, and demonic, strikes us irresistibly. But to succumb without understanding it, leads to fragmentation. This happens especially when the "demons" become absolutized as in superstition and aestheticism, where man is at the mercy of his passions and sentiments. It is therefore of utmost importance to destroy these fragmentizing tendencies. But to do so is to recognize them for what they are. This recognition is both spiritual nourishment ('food for thought') and the death of all which tends to starve man by preventing him from finding himself. In symbol representations Mahakala, the 'Black Lord of Transcending Awareness,' wields a flaming dagger with which to cut the thread of life of these demons, and holds a skull brimfull of their brain substance which he pours into his mouth.[30]

Most mad people do not have the presence of mind to be able to perform the religious medicine of sadhanas for themselves, so the lama can do it for them. This is a common prescription.

For neurotic people and people who are not totally incapacitated by their mental illness, it is strongly suggested that they perform as many religious practices as possible—as aspects of self-healing. Recitation of mantras is deemed especially beneficial for dispelling the demons of insanity from onself, but usually these are done while also taking special herbal psychiatric medicines. Meditation on equanimity, compassion, and love is strongly recommended.

There are also peaceful ways of propitiating the demons. One is to gently ask them to go away by offering pleasing things to them. These may be real or visualized offerings which are meant to satisfy them. It is a telling point to note that the offerings they are said to like best are our own defilements and attachments (which created them in the first place on a primordial level). When we can let go mentally in this way, they are satisfied. This means that our attachment to our habits, obscurations, aversions, and cravings is exactly what attracts these "ghosts." Our giving them up sends the ghosts away.

Other Dharma methods for dealing with them include, according to Patrul Rinpoche, confidence and devotion in the Buddha, in one's teachers and in the performance of mantras and rituals; performing charitable and virtuous activities; wearing blessed protection circles and charms as amulets; and taking special medicines especially prepared with mantras, applying mantra-blessed medicine butters to special points on the body and inhaling blessed medicinal incenses.

There are special incense and burnt offering rituals [*bsangs* and *gsur*] designed to satisfy all the different kinds of spirits, protectors and deities. Upon piles of fresh evergreen boughs consecrated mixtures of grains and foods (and sometimes medicinal herbs) are burned. The person doing the ritual visualizes the huge clouds of smoke that spiral skywards as being full of offering goddesses riding rainbow light beams and carrying oblations of everything that is both desired and needed. Through the power of visualization, the offerings are multiplied thousands-fold. One considers that all the spirits are satisfied and dissolve into rainbow light and then into the profound void space of the diamond-mind. It is said that Lama Mipham once wrote one of these offering rituals especially to allay an epidemic outbreak of mental illness in a particular part of Tibet and that he successfully pacified it with this practice.

Exorcism

Analysis of ritual exorcism in Tibetan Dharma reveals it to be the practice of active and pure spirituality rather than some magical hocus-pocus. Up until the last few decades, the Vajrayana and tantric Buddhism of Tibet was thought by most outsiders, scholars and even other kinds of Buddhists to be a sort of sorcery and priestcraft.

Especially in rites of exorcism and in anti-demonical measures the charges of idolatry and sacerdotalism found an easy target. But to the Tibetan Buddhists these rites and techniques are simply elaborate and tantric means of exercising the powers of wisdom and compassion. The form is magical in that it is the direct confronting and transforming of negative energies with means and awareness beyond limited rationality. Yet the lama-doctor-exorcist is a spiritual wizard who understands that he is purifying the demons of his own mind, as it were, the powerful "independent" forces of the unconscious as well as the negative forces in the outer world. He sees the demon to be the embodiment of negativity that is an inevitable

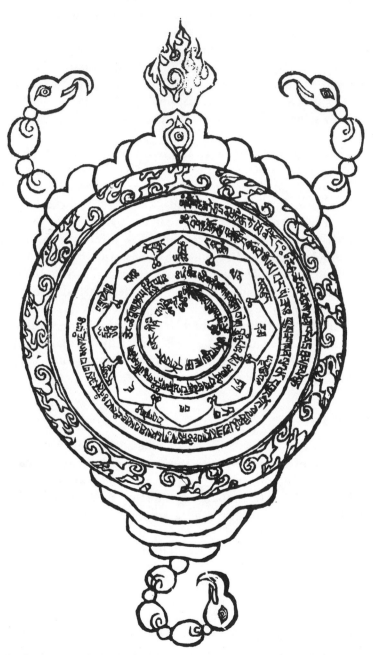

Figure 27 A scorpion charm with a protective mantric mandala especially used for warding off disease-causing demons. The name and birth sign of the person to be protected is filled in the empty space of the mandala; it can then be folded up and worn on the body as an amulet.

outcome of samsaric ignorance. He has compassion for ghosts and wishes to liberate them. There is no fear. The vajra nature of awareness-mind cannot be vitiated or defeated by ghosts or ideas of ghosts. Exorcism itself is not some spiritual weirdness draped in cruel and ritual veils (as it is pictured in the movies). It is a spiritual operation performed with the instruments of bodhiccita and compassion. As though in explication of this, the Tibetan scholar Giuseppi Tucci calls the great vajra master Padmasambhava "il exorcisti"—an apt title that expresses an essential element of tantra.

In the Tibetan tradition there are many types of ritual exorcism. Exorcism (*bgegs-bzlog-chog*) is a way of clearing away the demons, evil forces, and hindrances which are either obstructing Dharma practice or interfering with good health. If protective measures like mandala visualizations, mantras or amulets were not taken to prevent interference by demons, then the demons and spirits must be exorcised.

The first non-killing kind of exorcism is called ransoming (*glud*) the spirit. There are many varieties of this. One is that by making offerings and performing ritual *pujas,* the demons are satisfied and go away.

Another variety is the way of ransoming by effigy (*glud-tshab*). In this case an effigy of the sick person is made, usually of straw, and in it are placed many things such as pieces of the person's clothing, rice, sugar, salt, butter, and silver. This effigy is thrown in the direction from which the particular kind of spirit emanates. The demon is satisfied by this and goes away.

Another such method is that of the thread-cross ritual (*mdos*). A mastlike structure is created with colored threads which are said to be liked very, very much. (This looks like the Mexican "Eye-of-God".) It is put outside the house of the sick person and the demon is attracted to it and enters it—thereby accepting it as ransom.

The killing or threatening types of exorcisms are of three classes: by burying, by burning, by throwing. All of these as well as the above are accompanied by visualization and mantra which provide the motive power for the lama-doctor to successfully perform the exorcism. Further, in the destructive exorcisms, the consciousness of the demon is transferred by the lama to another realm in which it may hear Dharma and enter the path of liberation.

The threatening exorcism by means of burying (*mnan*) entails calling the spirits and making them enter something which is then buried.

Another wrathful method is by burning (*bsreg*). One way is to call them and then burn them in the hand with a special instrument. They are also attracted to sacrificial fire offerings—like melted butter which is placed in a container. The spirits enter it and are burned.

Another way of exorcism is by throwing (*'phang*). Here one makes something attractive to the spirits from dry grass. They are called to it and they enter it. Then a torma (offering-cake sculpture) is thrown onto it—heaved like a bomb. Then it is burned.[31]

For all of these kinds of exorcism there are two basic things needed: an understanding of emptiness and compassion for the spirits. If a person or a lama has these two, then there is really no need to perform elaborate rituals or exorcism. Emptiness and compassion are ultimate weapons and medicine.

Many times the lamas perform the exorcism simply because the patient and his family are very much impressed and attached to the ritual. The rite of exorcism helps the people by giving them a structure on which to see the negativity go away. This is similar, it is said, to projecting all your worries onto a rock and then throwing the rock away: it gives relief.

The Chod Rite

There is a special kind of offering used by advanced Dharma practitioners to pacify negative forces. It is called the chod (*gcod,* literally "cutting") ritual or the "mystic sacrifice" and involves developing wisdom, compassion and bodhicitta by cutting off one's sense of self as ego.

In essence, the person doing chod ritual calls all the negative spirits and offers his body to them. He invokes the host of elemental beings in order to subdue them (and himself). The rite is so powerful that the practitioner risks, according to Evans-Wentz, unbalanced psychic constitution, madness, or even death. This may be something of an exaggeration, but what Evans-Wentz implies is that one is confronting all the negative forces in oneself and one's world, and only according to the purity of one's spiritual intention, honesty, wisdom and compassion, will one be successful at offering one's ego to these beings, thereby liberating both them and oneself. Otherwise, they may well overwhelm the practitioner.

An obvious aspect of this mystic offering is that one's sense of ego-sense is intimately connected with attachment to the physical body. By visualizing, as one does in this practice, the body cut up into little pieces that are boiled in the cup of one's own skull, one breaks down ingrained attachment and clinging. So, in spite of the fact that the chod rite sounds terribly gory, sado-masochistic and cannibalistic, it is the precise opposite of those things. It is the cutting off of sensual attachment and egotism.

Chod is a way of liberation that expands awareness for the well-being of others, according to Ma-Chig-La, the female lama who was among its greatest propagators in Tibet. And, in fact, the practice of the mystic sacrifice can render the practitioner supremely capable of benefiting others. For example, the story is told of a certain monastery in Tibet devoted to the practice of chod, and when an epidemic of cholera broke out in this area, the monks could be seen going everywhere attending the sick and carrying away the dead. Because they had no attachment to their bodies and hence no fear, they could serve the needs of others without hesitation.

The practice of chod is performed in meditation. Making prayers to realize the wisdom-mind of the pure Dharmakaya and being resolved before the lineage of gurus to conquer delusion in oneself, one performs the sacrifice of one's own body. First it is visualized as being fat and ugly, the hook on which we hang our hates and lusts and ego. Then one imagines a wrathful wisdom goddess standing apart from it; she represents one's own inherent wisdom-nature. She cuts off our head and flings bits of our body into our skull, which is set boiling as a cauldron. It radiates inconceivable offerings of light.

The light rays become different offerings appropriate for the "four guests": the Three Jewels, the protectors, sentient beings, and the various spirits. One imagines that the handicapped, the hungry, the poor, the sick and the lonely, etc. etc. arrive to receive whatever they need—eyes, limbs, food, wealth, comfort, care. The demons, too, receive in the form of light whatever quells their torment and aggression.

At the end of the practice, after the dedication of merit, there may follow a prayer of aspiration to be fulfilled when the practitioner becomes enlightened.

> May all of you (unenlightened spirits and elementals) be born [as humans] and become my first disciples.
>
> Thereupon, may the Uncreated Essence of the Pure, Unborn Mind
>
> Arise in the nature of the three—deities, men and elementals;

And, avoiding the path of the misleading belief in the
reality of the "I"

May their principle of consciousness be thoroughly
saturated with the moisture of Love and Compassion.[32]

Summary

All the means and techniques for expelling demons—mantras,
visualizations of protective circles, devotion to the deity, exorcisms of
various kinds—are in essence different expressions of the ultimate
medicines: compassion and emptiness. These are the two great
powers, the two great meditations, that subdue all diseases and evil
spirits.

"Ghosts," negative thought forms, evil energies, "demons,"
harmful spirits, etc. are the names and forms which the Tibetan
system has given to those dark forces which influence us, overtake us
and possess us so that we no longer act and think in a manner which is
harmonious with our deepest coherence of being. In other words, we
become insane, self-destructive, not really ourselves.

Such forces span a large range from the purely psychological—
our own demons, so to speak—to the cosmic forces which attack us
in accordance with larger laws of karma.

Their numbers, types, and qualities are the way in which a highly
developed system of classification of mental illness is expressed in the
Tibetan system.

These "ghosts" and "demons" are a shared symbolic language
which is rich in meaning to the members of the community and
something that the Tibetan people relate to very vividly.

The variety of negative forces and demons causing various kinds
of madness and mental disease mirror the variety of distinct
psychopathology expressed in the Tibetan system. As such they offer
rich material for psychological interpretation and for ways of viewing
psychosis.

10

Three Psychiatric Chapters Translated from the Gyu-Zhi

These psychiatric chapters from the *Gyu-zhi* represent what is perhaps the oldest written and complete tradition of medical psychiatry in the world, more than a thousand years old and still surviving in the twentieth century, preserved by unbroken lineages of Tibetans.

As we have seen, these texts date from at least the eighth century in India, when the *Gyu-zhi* was translated and brought to Tibet where it was redacted in the eleventh century. The entire *Gyu-zhi* echoes the earliest existent classic works of Indian Ayurveda. In these chapters the names of some of the "demons" come from the Indian tradition. In the *Charaka Samhita,* where one can find some lines and prescriptions that are almost exactly the same, there are only seven demons listed in the one chapter on insanity as opposed to eighteen elemental spirits and two other types of demons in the three chapters here.

For example, regarding psychiatry Charaka says that insanity can be explained either (constitutionally) as a disturbance of the organism—the "incensed" humors overflowing into the special canals which carry "the subtle mind stuff" or (accidentally) by an influx of super human powers (demons) brought on by "hostile, inharmonious, vitiated or impure attacks on deities, Brahmans, seniors. . . mental shock caused by fear and joy. . . abnormal efforts" and also wrong food.[33] These basic ideas are found in the *Gyu-zhi,* but

what we have in the Tibetan text is a much more developed and
sophisticated system, and one that has living masters to explicate and
practice it.

In a concise way these chapters reveal the full range of Tibetan
psychiatry: a refined system of etiology and diagnosis based on
definite symptoms—the character and behavior of the kinds of

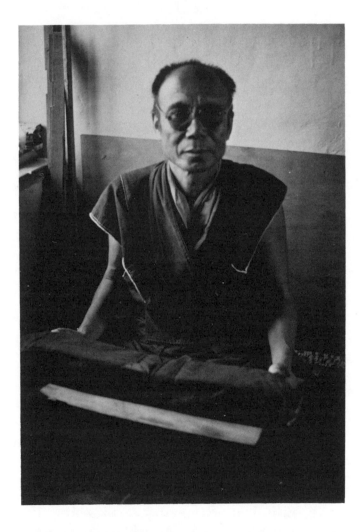

Figure 28 Lama Dodrag Amchi (*amchi* means doctor) of Kedrup Sherab Ling
Monastery in Nepal. He is holding a copy of the *Gyu-zhi* in his lap, its long unbound
pages wrapped in cloth in the traditional manner. Amchi-la explained the *Gyu-zhi's*
three chapters on mental illness.

"demons" as well as a variety of somatic and psychological symptoms—and an elaborate system of treatment with herbal and spiritual medicines that attacks all levels of the disorder.

All the elements of Tibetan Buddhist medicine are involved in these three chapters on psychiatry. We have already discussed all the elements individually. Now we will find them coherently organized together in these psychiatric texts.

The texts are extremely abbreviated. In some cases just one syllable in the text is enough to indicate a whole religious or medical teaching. These would be basically unintelligible and untranslatable without the guidance of a lama or doctor to explicate their meaning. This has been done by Lama Dodrag Amchi of Bodhanath, Nepal; the notes that follow the translation of each chapter come primarily from his comments.

The following three chapters of the Third Tantra called the "Pith Instructions" (*Man-ngag-rgyud*) of the *Gyu-zhi* represent the heart of the Tibetan medical psychiatric tradition. They are in the form of a dialogue between the rishi Rigpai Yeshe, an emanation of the mind of the Medicine Buddha, and the sage Yilay Kye, an emanation of the speech of the Medicine Buddha.

CHAPTERS 77, 78 AND 79

OF

THE THIRD TANTRA

THE MAN-NGAG-RGYUD

THE PITH INSTRUCTIONS

OF

THE RGYUD-BZHI

Translated[34] from a reproduction of a set of prints from the 18th century *Zung-cu-ze* blocks from the collection of Raghu Vira, published by S.W. Tashigang, 1975, Leh, Ledakh.

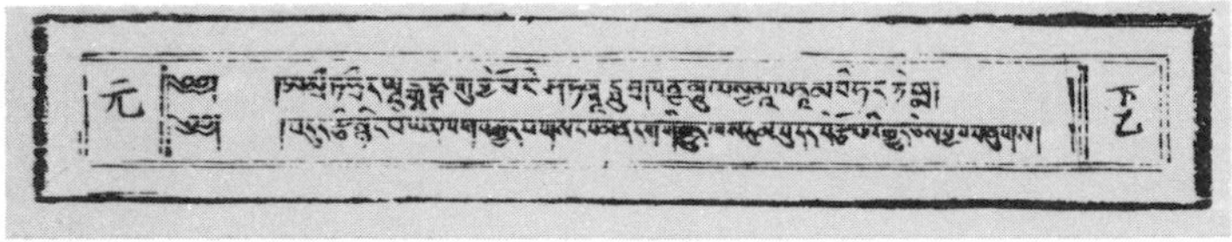

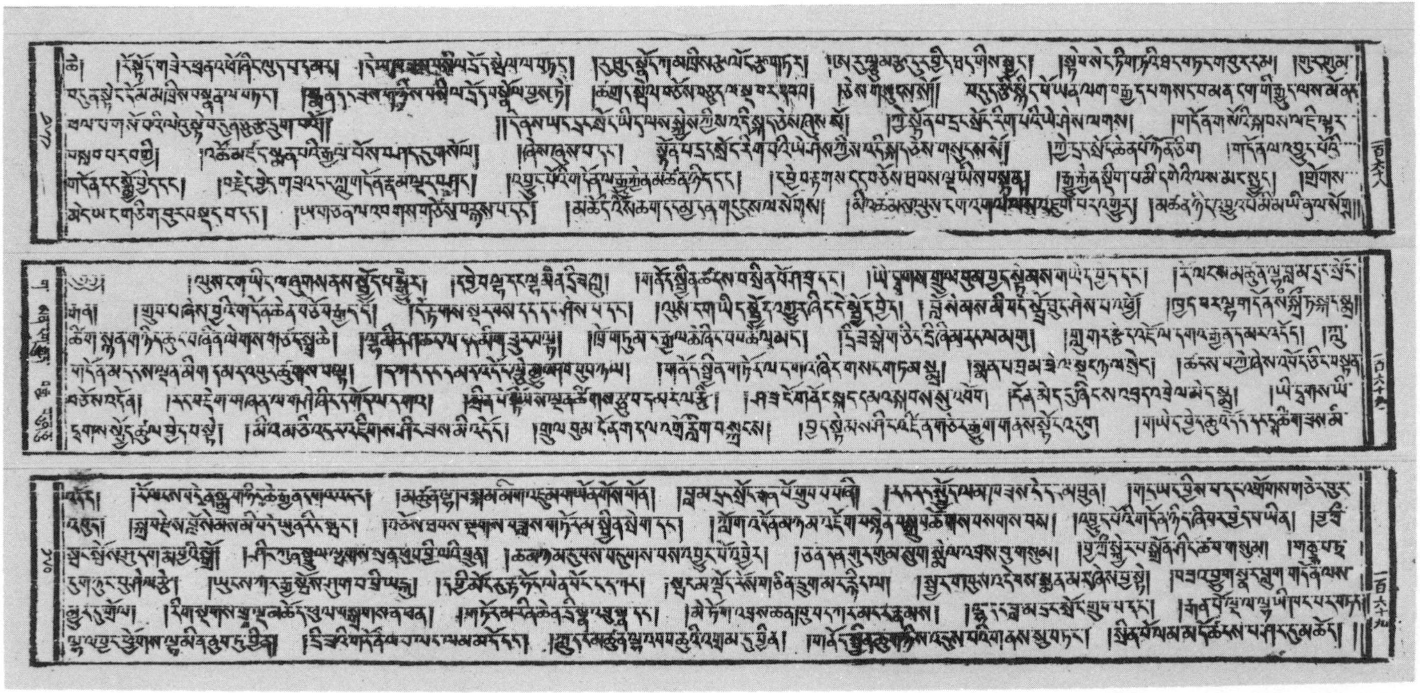

Figure 29 The smallest folio is the title page of the *Gyu-zhi*, the thousand year old Tibetan medical work. The rest of the folios shown here are reproductions of the original text discussed in this chapter.

Chapter 77

Chapter 77 enumerates eighteen separate "elemental spirits" (*'byung-po'i gdon*) that cause a sudden type of insanity. These elemental spirits have peculiar traits and characteristics that are expressed as psychopathology in the human beings affected or "possessed" by them. The classification of the elemental spirits, then, is a classification of eighteen varieties of psychoses.

Each of the eighteen elemental spirits is named after a higher type of god, force, demon, or human whose behavior is imitated in the psychopathology of the patient. In the text, the names of the higher gods, demons, etc. are affixed with a grammatical term for the possessive case and then with the word *gdon,* meaning negative force, radiating effect or demon.

Thus, the first elemental spirit is named *lha'i gdon,* which means the demonic effect of the gods, the ghost of the gods, god-demons, or the negative effect of the gods. That is to say that the person is not possessed by the gods but by a negative force that causes him to behave in a manner reminiscent of the gods.

The question of whether the negative effects of the elementals arise from within the patient's own mind or whether they come from outside is not addressed in the text. However, they are all archetypal forms of negativity that suddenly overtake consciousness and thus provoke insane behavior very different from the patient's normal mode of action.

Each of the eighteen elemental spirits is listed below.

1. *Lha. Gods.* The whole class of minor gods from the upper regions of samsara. Gods (*devas*) form one of the six main divisions of the wheel of life; they are full of pride and have long pleasurable lives. *Lha'i gdon*: demonic effect of the gods.

2. *Lha-min. Jealous Gods* (*asuras*). The anti- or jealous gods, although they have a high position in the wheel of life, are entirely consumed with jealousy of the higher gods, whom they are always attacking. Their bodies are half god and half animal. They are said to live on the banks of the great ocean that surrounds Mt. Meru, the center of the universe where the gods live. A measure of the constant state of anxiety in which they exist is that they spend their time carving huge vats of wood to empty out the ocean that they fear will imminently overflow. *Lha-min-gyi gdon*: demonic effect of the jealous gods.

3. *Dri-za. Scent Eaters* (*gandarvas*). They come from the zone of

scents. They are attracted to sweet smelling things, but also to dung hills and other foul smelling places. *Dri-za'i gdon*: demonic effect of the scent eaters.

4. *kLu. Serpent-Spirits (nagas).* They have serpent bodies with human heads. They live in water and trees. The deities among them guard great Dharma treasures beneath the ocean. They are extremely powerful and dangerous when angry. *kLu'i gdon*: demonic effect of the serpent-spirits.

5. *gNod-sbyin. Harm-Givers (yakshas).* They haunt mountain passes and similar places and are sometimes called direction-demons. Travelers are advised to make offerings to them, for they often cause harm. *gNod-sbyin-gyi gdon*: demonic effect of the harm-givers.

6. *Tshangs-pa. Pervasive Spirit (Brahma).* Brahma is the Hindu Supreme Being, "pervasive holiness." *Tshangs-pa'i gdon*: demonic effect of pervasive holiness.

7. *Srin-po. Cannibal Spirits (rakshas).* Gargantuan red-eyed, red-necked cannibal-spirits who go about at night and harm humans. Guru Padmasambhava subdued them in Tibet. *Srin-po'i gdon*: demonic effect of the cannibal spirits.

8. *Sha-za. Flesh-Eater Spirits.* These are invisible eaters of human meat and blood. *Sha-za'i gdon*: demonic effect of the flesh-eater spirits.

9. *Yi-dags. Hungry Ghosts.* These are one of the six major divisions of beings in the wheel of life. Beings are reborn in that realm due to extreme greed. They have huge bloated stomachs and thin parched throats. They are tormented by constant and insatiable want of food and drink which, even if they find, they are unable to ingest. *Yi-dags-kyi gdon*: demonic effect of hungry ghosts.

10. *Grul-bum. Vampire Ghouls.* They live in cemeteries and cremation grounds and drink blood. *Grul-bum-gi gdon*: demonic effect of vampire ghouls.

11. *Byad-stems. Evil-Curse Ghosts.* These are negative spirit forms created by humans and sent to harm an enemy. *Byad-stems-kyi gdon*: demonic effect of evil curse ghosts.

12. *Yeng-ched. Mental Agitators.* Spirits of distractions who disturb the mental process, especially memory, and who produce inattention and mindlessness. *Yeng-ched-kyi gdon*: demonic effect of mental agitators.

13. *Ro-langs. Zombies.* A dead body infused with an evil spirit. Some cannot bend from the waist; they have enormous strength. *Ro-langs-kyi gdon*: demonic effect of zombies.

14. *mTshun-lha. Ancestor Gods.* The original household gods of the Tibetan shamans. The spirits of the ancestral lineage. *mTshun-lha-yi gdon*: demonic effect of ancestor gods.

15. *bLa-ma. Guru.* A spiritual teacher, guru, lama or mentor. *bLa-ma'i gdon*: demonic effect in the manner of a guru. The demon behaves in the manner of a spiritual teacher and likes to perform pujas, etc.

16. *Drang-srong. Sage. Drang-srong-gi gdon*: demonic effect of sages. The demon adopts the manner of rishis, sages who dress in white and have great wisdom, like to stay alone and keep very clean.

17. *rGan-po. Respected Elder.* They are old, pure in learning and manner, have the posture of old men, and prefer quiet places. *rGan-po'i gdon*: demonic effect of respected elders.

18. *Grub-pa. Magical Emanation.* This is a magical emanation created by a siddha, one who has accomplished tantric powers by the power of his tantric practice. *Grub-pa'i gdon*: demonic effect of magical emanations (or the actual siddhas).

These are the eighteen "great elementals" from among all elemental spirits. The first one and the last four of them, that is, the god-demon, the guru (lama) demon, the sage demon, the respected elder demon and the accomplishment emanation demon, form a separate category known as the five highest elementals.

These five are said to be like seeds—the seeds of future madness and possession; the body is the land where they are planted. The eighteen great elemental spirits, in general, are like the farmers who nourish the seed and bring it to fruition. Madness and possession by elementals cannot come out of this order.[35]

Chapter 77 describes how people who are possessed by these elementals act mad in accordance with the particular demon's disposition, behavior and cravings. The descriptions are brief but highly evocative. They often correspond to classical symptoms and types of psychopathology as described in Western psychiatry.

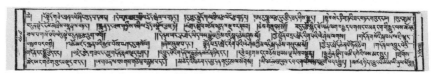

Figure 30 Chapters do not begin on separate pages. Chapter 77 begins after the large space in the third line of the folio shown here. This and the ones that follow are reductions of the folios shown in figure 29.

The 77th Chapter of the Third Tantra of Pith Instructions:

ELEMENTAL SPIRITS

Then the sage Yilay Kye asked as follows: O great rishi Rigpai Yeshe, do speak of the way to cure all evil spirits [*gdon*] who cause disease. Pray let the King of Medicine who sustains life explain. He requested thusly.

The teacher Rigpai Yeshe spoke as follows: O great sage, harken.

Evil spirits are explained in five groups: elemental spirits, madness-causing demons; amnesia-causing demons; planetary-spirits [causing epilepsy]; and serpent-spirit demons [causing leprosy].

Regarding the elemental spirits, the teaching is five-fold: Cause; character; class; symptom; and cure.

The Cause:[a] Performing many sins and unvirtuous actions; sitting alone without even a single friend;[b] defiling, harming, and despising the demon's place;[c] going against what is worthy of honor;[d] and being tormented by sorrow;[e] etc. [In short] entering into improper physical and spoken action opposed to law.

The Characteristics: The non-human elemental spirits reside in one's body, speech and mind and control one's behavior.

The Classes: The eighteen great classes of elemental spirits are called: god-demons; anti-god demons; scent-eater demons; serpent-spirit demons; harm-giver demons; pervasive-spirit demons; cannibal-demons; flesh-eater demons; hungry-ghost demons; vampire-ghoul demons; evil-curse spirit demons; mental-agitator demons; zombie demons; ancestor-spirit demons; guru demons; sage demons; respected-elder demons; and accomplishment-emanation demons.

The Symptoms: These elemental spirits possess one's body, speech, and mind and commit one's acts. One's mind becomes unhappy, and consciousness wavers restlessly.

In particular [people possessed by] the demonic effect of the gods speak Sanskrit[f] and sweet words, sleep little, are good natured, and keep very clean.

[People possessed by] the demonic effect of the anti-gods like meat and wine, look indirectly out of the corners of their eyes, and speak much reckless talk. They have great pride and fierce anger.

[People possessed by] the effect of the scent-eaters are graceful and delight in fragrant smells. They like to sing, dance, and play. They love to wear nice clothes and are attracted towards red ornaments.

[People possessed by] the demonic effect of the serpent spirits have radiant faces and red bloodshot eyes with straight piercing stares. They desire the whites [curds, milk, and butter] and the reds [meat]. They flick their tongues and sleep face downward.[g]

[People possessed by] the effect of the harm givers like offering cakes [torma] and fish. They tell secrets[h] and hate doctors and holy people.

[People possessed by] the demonic effect of pervasive holiness cry out the name of God and expound on religious scriptures. They beat themselves, abuse others, and like to laugh.

[People possessed by] the demonic effect of the cannibal demons possess great physical strength, talk roughly, and like meat.

[People possessed by] the demonic effect of the invisible flesh-eaters are ashamed of themselves—they have low voices and downcast manner. They faint without reason and talk disjointedly; they scratch at the earth and fields.

[People possessed by] the demonic effect of the hungry ghosts act according to the mode of action of hungry ghosts.[i]

[People possessed by] the demonic effect of ugly evil ghosts[j] quake with fear and have no desire for food.

[People possessed by] the demonic effect of vampire ghouls have dark faces, walk slowly, and have swelling on their genitals.

[People possessed by] the demonic effect of evil curse ghosts like to carry wood,[k] go naked, and sit in solitary places.

[People possessed by] the demonic effect of the mental agitators drink much water, speak suddenly then stop, and do not like food.

[People possessed by] the demonic effect of the zombies speak the straight truth, sleep much, like ornaments, and have shaking bodies.

[People possessed by] the demonic effect of the ancestral spirits have dry mouths and squinting eyes. They wear their clothes backwards.[l]

[People possessed by] the demonic effects of the guru, the sage, the respected-elder, and the accomplished emanation are all consistent in their paths of action and diet.[m] They befriend all children, go naked, and cannot stay in one place. They have wild hair, unhappy minds, and feel long abandoned.

The Cure:[n] The nature of elemental spirits is pacified by recitation of mantra, offering cakes, burnt offering,[o] reading scriptures, meditation, sadhana,[p] service, and accumulation of "tshog."[q]

The elemental spirits are expelled by burning incense made from equal proportions of the following:[r]

valerian
Bya-kri
sweet flag rhizome
peacock's feathers [actual peacock feathers and a grass by that name]
asafoetida
pease-straw
black cat's feces
snake skin.

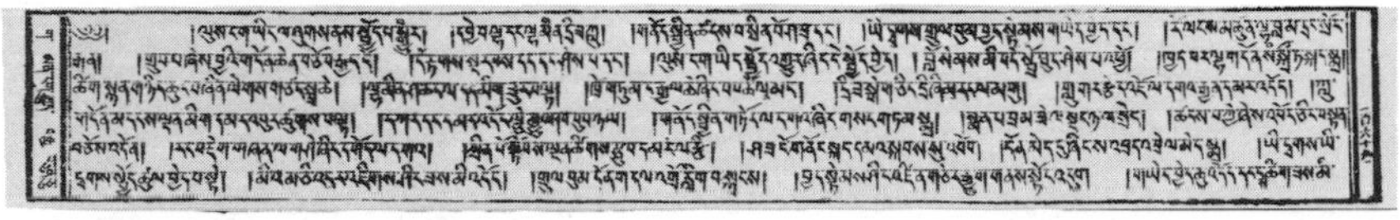

Figure 31 Chapter 77 describes the psychoses caused by elemental spirits.

All these elemental spirits are swiftly liberated by the use of an edible ointment and snuff called "medicine butter." It is compounded of:

the three chief fruits [Chebulic myrobalan—*arura*, Beleric myrobalan, Emblic myrobalan]
sandalwood
saffron crocus
bya-kri
the three hots [ginger, long pepper, black pepper]
cardamon
barberry
pine
Fanacetum sibiricum
Holarrhena antidysenterica
pu-shel-rtsi [khus-khus or orchid]
white mustard
Indian valerian

juniper
lavender
Piper chaba
Costus speciosus
hellebore
white aconite
spang-ma
realgar
the "six urines."[s]

It helps if [the above] is accompanied by worshipful offerings, and [the use of] the five paths of mantric science.[t]

Put offering cakes, gems and precious substances, perfumes, wheat and grains, flowers, cooked milk-rice, juice [or tea, etc.], the whites [milk, curds, butter], and the sweets [molasses, white sugar, honey] for the five [major] demons—gods, mentor, sage, elder, and accomplished emanation—at the places where they reside.

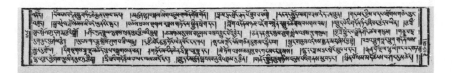

Figure 32   The continuation of Chapter 77, describing how to dispel the schizophrenic effects caused by "demons."

Offer[u] to the demons of the gods in the northern direction and to the anti-gods in the western direction. Offer to the scent-eaters at crossroads and cowsheds; to water-serpents and the ancestral spirits at river banks and waterfalls. Put the offerings for the harm-giving demons at the place where two streams of water meet, and for the cannibal demons at crossroads. Honor the pervasive-spirit demons at the eastern direction; put [offerings] for the flesh-eater demons in deserted houses in the western direction.

At the time when the elementals take hold on their own, especially rely upon [procedures] such as medicinal incense, offering cakes, and fire offerings.

Thus he spoke.

Here ends the seventy-seventh chapter on curing elemental spirits from the tantra of profound secret instruction, the eight branched essential nectar.

Chapter 77—Notes

a. The seed was already planted. These causes "water" it and bring it to fruition.

b. Especially at places like cemeteries and other deserted quiet spots.

c. Ghosts and demons have places—some in trees, others in water. Behavior which demeans and defiles the ghost's environment causes a bad reaction.

d. Breaking promises, breaking samaya vows with lama and deity, and breaking, for example, the bond over which the ghost rules, i.e., not propitiating the gods and ancestors, then they become angry and attack.

e. Sadness over emotional ties, i.e., fighting with spouse, or any emotional stress and strain, or, more basically, from experiencing impermanence and emptiness with attachment.

f. Sanskrit is the archetypal holy language in the East. Manifestation in the West could be in any sacred language along with similar religious preoccupations.

g. In the manner of a snake, face and body are straight and facing downwards in sleep.

h. Or—"they talk to themselves."

i. They are tormented by ravenous appetites for food and drink which can never be satisfied.

j. Not on the list of the eighteen, but, in general, it is a ghost in the more limited Western sense of the spirit of a dead person.

k. Or similar heavy loads and fondness for such work.

l. Literally "wear their robes on the left side." That is, reversed from the right way in which the monastic robe is always worn.

m. Act and eat in conformity with their types; see introductory list.

n. These satisfy the various desires of the ghosts so then they don't need to bother people.

o. Incense offerings are especially good for pacification; see previous explanation.

p. Especially the sadhanas (ritual practice) of Chenrezi, the embodiment of compassion, and Vajrapani, the embodiment of power and the subduer of evil spirits.

q. An assemblage of large and varied offerings used in special tantric practices.

r. For this medicine and the others to follow the spiritual state of mind of the doctor is crucial. One must consider all ingredients as being very clean and pure. One must do puja and blessings for the medicines. One should not tell the patient what is in the medicine. This medicine is mixed and ground until it is almost dust. Then a pinch of it is burned on coals and the patient inhales it; a cloth on his head covers the incense so all is inhaled.

s.   Urine was used as a medicine extensively in Ayurveda, especially for mental diseases.

t.   As described by Lord Buddha and recorded in the Kanjur.

u.   Like the preceding offering.

Chapter 78

Chapter 78 deals with a kind of madness called "nyo" (*smyo*) which is related to the senses, to emotional and organic disturbances of a psychiatric nature as opposed to the abrupt splits in consciousness of the previous chapter.

The causes of madness are enumerated in seven classes. In six out of seven cases it is organic and emotional factors which are the primary causes of madness. In those cases the emotional and organic disturbances are the direct development of the patient's humoral and mental disposition, unlike the situation described in Chapter 77 where the elemental spirits produce sudden symptoms very different from the patient's normal disposition. The exception here is the seventh case where the madness-causing demon (*smyo-byed-kyi gdon*) acts alone.

An essential difference between the ghosts of Chapter 77 and the demons of Chapter 78 is that the former all have distinct character and behavioral traits, while the latter are more general spirits of madness that goad the senses and the emotions.

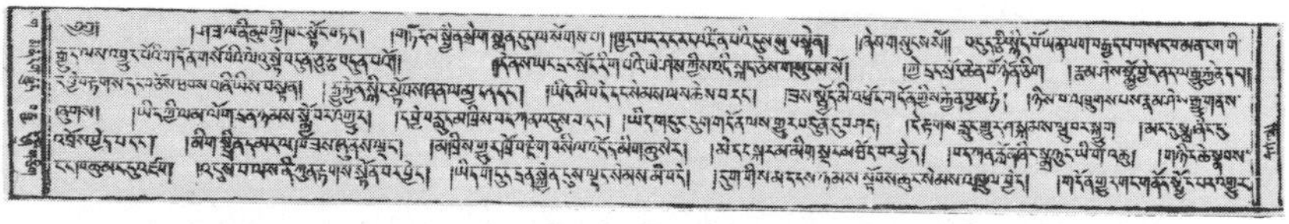

Figure 33 Chapter 78 begins on the second line of this folio; it describes the causes and symptoms of madness.

The 78th Chapter of the Third Tantra of Pith Instructions:

MADNESS-CAUSING GHOSTS

Then the rishi Rigpai Yeshe spoke as follows: O great sage, harken.

The illness which makes consciousness insane is taught in four [parts]: Cause, class, symptom, and cure.

The Cause: Feeble heart power,[a] depression, unhappy mind, anxious over-thinking,[b] and unwholesome diet [are the primary causes which] assist the secondary cause—demons.

Secondarily, the mental confusion causes consciousness to stay in the place of the path of mind, perverting it so that recollection becomes dim and one becomes insane.[c]

Class: It [madness] is explained in seven classes: madness arising from vital wind; from bile; from phlegm; from a combination of those three; from distressed mind; from poison; and from ghosts.

The Symptoms: Arising from wind, the flesh becomes emaciated, one vomits foam, talks and cries much and runs about hither and dither. The eyes are red and cloudy and [the illness] gets worse after taking food.

Arising from bile, one becomes angry and violent, likes the cold, has yellow tears, and sees fire and stars before the eyes.

[Arising] from phlegm, one becomes damp, speaks little, has revulsion to food, sleeps a lot and has much mucus dripping from the nose and much saliva trickling out of the mouth.

[Arising] from a combination [of the humors], all the symptoms are revealed.

[Arising] from mental distress, one is all the time thinking of one's sadness.[d]

[Arising] from poison, the mind becomes confused, the radiance of the face is greatly diminished, and there is little bodily vigor.[e]

[Arising] from a demonic force all conduct becomes harmful.

The Cure: There are two methods [of cure]: the general and the particular.

First in order to clear the openings where the mind enters,[f] purify by ointment massage[g] [*bsku-mnye*], by medicinal bath,[h] by forced vomiting and by letting blood.[i]

[Then] use the medicine called "the virtuous medicine butter" [which consists of]:

old butter
the three chief fruits [Chebulic myrobalan—*arura,* Beleric myrobalan, Emblic myrobalan]
Vitex agnus-castus
pine
sarsaparilla
turmeric
barberry
Desmodium gangeticum
Indian valerian
Costus speciosus
raspberry [or salamin]
lavender
cobra's saffron
rhododendron
purging cassia
pomegranate
Erycibe paniculata
cubeb
Piper chaba
blue lotus
sandalwood
juniper.

It[j] [virtuous medicine butter] engenders strong sexual drive and potency, the conception of a child, a strong body, and the complete uprooting of the causes of insanity.

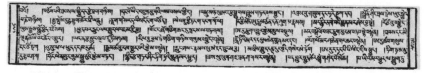

Figure 34 Chapter 78 continues with the various medicine formulas for treating insanity.

In particular, for a problem arising from the vital air rely upon the mild purgative medicine called "Gentle Juices" ['*jam-rtsi*]: Grind one dram of aconite with strong beer. Then combine it with six drams of myrobalan until it becomes a powder, then mix it with water. Rely upon mixing this with butter, molasses, and the "six good things" [cardamon, cubeb, nutmeg, bamboo pith, cloves and saffron]. Without the proper method [this medicine] can become an obstacle to life.[k]

Or else rely upon one, two or three pills of equal amounts of nutmeg and the five garudas [myrobalan, *Costus speciosus,* sweet flag rhizome, cloves and sandalwood].

[Or] compound a powder mixture of:
    molasses
    sea salt
    black salt
    bishop's weed
    coriander
    tsi-tra-ka (capsicum or leadwort)
    the three hots [ginger, black pepper, long pepper]
    myrobalan.

[Or] compound:
    nutmeg
    butter
    human bones
    medicine butter
    human [or animal] meat dried for one year
    strong beer.

The "burning spoon"[l] [herbal moxibustion] should be applied on all the secret [points for the] vital airs.[m]

For disturbances in bile, first purify by mixing:[n]

    long pepper
    chebulic myrobalan
    yellow champa
    castor oil plant
    blue lotus root.

[Then] make a powder[o] of:
    gentian
    elecampane
    Adhatoda vasica
    hellebore
    saffron crocus
    emblic myrobalan

Let blood from the heart vein.[P] Mix gentian into medicine butter; and rely upon taking the fresh meat of sheep and beef for food.

For disturbance of phlegm induce vomiting with a mixture[q] of:
    cow's milk
    ginger
    Sebania grandiflora
    plumeless thistle.

And rely upon powerful nourishment[r] and "burning spoon"[s] medicine.

For a disturbance due to the combination [of the three humors], we should compound the cures for all.

Cure the distressed mind by the wealth of Dharma and with the help of sweet talk.

For disturbance from poison, rely upon a tablet made of:
    dpa-ser
    white aconite
    red aconite
    re-ral
    turmeric
    "fragrant water" [urine][t].

For change due to spirits,[u] burn the incense mixture of the urine, feces, bile, nails, hair, and skin of:
    cat
    ram
    owl
    fox.

Thus it was said.

[Here ends] the seventh-eighth chapter on curing the ghosts which cause insanity from the tantra of profound secret instruction, the eight branched essential nectar.

Chapter 78—Notes

a. Not necessarily a physical heart disorder, but heart-sickness associated with sleeplessness, starvation, despair, etc. and weakness of the heart-center which affects the winds.
b. Intellectual and conceptual preoccupation with anxiety-ridden thoughts.
c. The path of mind is the normal flowing of the energies of the five skandhas through the five veins of consciousness. Here

it is blocked and perverted at the crucial space at the center of the heart where all the veins meet.

There are "six gates" or veins of sense consciousness branching off the first vein of sense consciousness meeting at that space as well.

According to various systems, the six gates and the channels of consciousness at the heart center are described in slightly different ways.

In the *Lapis Lazuli* commentary it is explained that in the middle of the heart chakra there are eight petals surrounding the central column. In the heart there are four nerves (four main petals) going in the four directions and also one going up and one going down. These are the "six gates."

The one going in the upward direction is green and is the path of body consciousness. Downward direction is blue and is thought consciousness. Eastward (in front) is black and ear consciousness. South (right side) is red and eye consciousness. West (back) is yellow and nose consciousness. North (left) is white and is tongue consciousness.

Ghosts enter from the eastern and downward direction. They come in with confused and agitated thinking, insert into the vital space and stay there, perverting the path of mind.

d. For example, one loses his or her spouse and dwells upon this and so the sadness increases and makes mental trouble arise; a closed circuit of neurotic thoughts which repeat themselves and become stronger and stronger.

e. Even good nourishment and essences don't bring the body back to health in the case of madness by poison. The mind remains immersed in illusion.

f. Pores or openings (*bu-ga*). Not only the inner channels but also the outer pores of skin (skin is related to mind in Tibetan medicine) can, when blocked, adversely affect the mental functioning. If air can pass properly, then mind functions smoothly.

g. These are preliminary purification treatments: massage for wind; purge with vomiting for phlegm; bath for bile; bloodletting for blood (sometimes classified as a fourth humor).

h. This special medicinal bath for bile is called the Bath of the Five Nectars (*bDud-rtsi lnga-lums*). It contains:
   Tibetan tamarisk
   dwarf rhododendhron
   juniper

Tenacetum tomentosum—an aromatic plant
an evergreen grass.

To these are added here two main anti-air herbs, nutmeg and
cloves, since air is disturbed in all psychiatric cases. All these are
used in equal amounts and closed in an air-tight pot for fifteen
days; then they are put in bath water where they ferment.

i. Let blood from big toe and fingers. Some kinds of hot and bile
    madness are associated with an abundance of blood. "Let blood"
    also includes checking the subtle veins.

j. Difficult to prepare. First these are pounded into powder then
    boiled as a soup. Ratio is 1 powder to 6 milk and 3 old butter
    which are all boiled together as a soup for two days or so, until it
    becomes very clear. Then it is kept in a cold place until it becomes
    butter. One spoonful in morning and evening.

k. This powerful medicine is taken in small doses—here orally. In
    the Fourth Tantra it is prescribed as an enema. Too much is
    deadly.

l. *"Me dang thur-ma."* Literally fire and spoon, which means
    moxibustion. The spoon is iron, gold, or copper needles. *Thur-ma*
    also is the name of the grass medicine used in the moxibustion (a
    grass *spra*).

m. The spots for moxa here are the base of the neck and the sixth
    vertebra down from the base of the neck (seventh cervical and
    fourth thoracic), and the xiphisternal notch.

n. These are made into powder and given as preliminary medicine
    when the patient has bad digestion.

o. Eat one spoon of the powder in the afternoon with hot water. For
    bile types medicines must be given in the afternoon and evening.

p. In the arch of the foot.

q. These are boiled and eaten. The phlegm sickness comes out with
    vomiting.

r. Proper anti-phlegm foods such as brown flour, vegetables, corn,
    soybeans, and animal organs—stomach, etc.—but not fresh
    animal flesh.

s. For phlegm the spots are on mid-stomach and on third vertebra
    down from base of neck—first thoracic.

t. Mix the powder of the above with red cow's urine. The cow must
    have been inside a house for seven days and should have had clean
    grass to eat. The urine should be taken at sunrise, then strained
    and then boiled with the powder until it yields a thick paste.

Urine, especially that of a healthy and clean person or animal, is believed to be an excellent antiseptic and anti-toxin. It can be applied directly to an open wound to prevent infection if nothing else is available. Here it is used to counter an internal toxic reaction.

u. No disturbance of the humors, poisons or emotion, only the madness ghost is strong here. This madness ghost has no strong personality characteristic of its own, unlike the elementals in the previous chapter.

Chapter 79

The category and manner of operation of the demons who cause oblivion (*brjed-byed-kyi gdon*) of Chapter 79 are very similar to the demons who cause madness of the previous chapter. Basically only their effect is different.

Whereas those of Chapter 78 have a poisonous emotional effect, a sort of goading of the senses, these of Chapter 79 radiate an effect on mental functioning, particularly the memory function—its disturbances, dysfunction, and loss. They drain their victims of the ability to concentrate, effect a loss of sensibility and, in the extreme, a complete loss of memory.

Both these groups of demons are specifically linked with organic and psychological imbalances which are the primary causes of the illness in all but one case and which permit the demons to overtake their victims. The one exception is where the demon operates alone. The cases in both chapters where the demon does not operate alone provide the basic theory and treatment of organic and psychological causes of psychopathology. These can and often are interpreted as being independent of demons since the demon is the secondary effect in consequence of other factors.

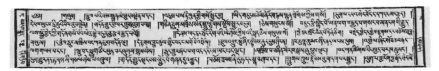

Figure 35 Chapter 79 begins on the third line of this folio; it describes types of dementia and memory loss.

The 79th Chapter of the Third Tantra of Pith Instruction:

THE SPIRITS WHO CAUSE FORGETFULNESS

Then the rishi Rigpai Yeshe spoke these words: O great sage, harken.

The causes of oblivion are [explained] in three [parts]: Class, symptoms, and method of cure.

The Class: There are five classes: life wind, bile, phlegm, poison, and spirits.

The Symptoms: Palpitations of the heart, dizziness in the head,[a] bloated stomach, decreased vigor, aching spine,[b] much oral spittle, and nasal mucus at the time the sickness arises; also, fainting, grinding teeth, shaking of the hands and feet, vomiting of foam; and all thought is lost in darkness.[c]

Arising from the life wind there is quaking of hands and feet; and agitated getting up and down again and again.[d]

Arising from bile the complexion becomes yellow and the mouth dry; [the sickness is] worse at mealtimes.[e]

Arising from phlegm the joints are swollen and there is especially much saliva.

Arising from poison, the symptoms of the sickness are unclear [and there are] hallucinations.[f]

Arising from demons, one's conduct becomes other than before.[g]

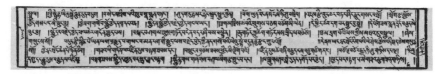

Figure 36 The conclusion of Chapter 79.

The Method of Cure: Purify the orifices with acrid washes for vomiting, nasal purges, and medicinal enemas.[h]

Burn incense smoke from:

owl [feather]
crow [feather]
vulture [feather]
zermo [feather]

snake [skin and meat]
dog [feces]
monkey [feces]
horse [feces].

Put medicine made from the bile of a yellow cow up the nose.[i]
Offer a medicine of:

sweet flag rhizome
Costus speciosus
old butter
honey.

If [the person had] fallen down unconscious for a long time, burn twenty-five [points] on the fingers and toes.[j]

Having given a mild purgative of strong beer,[k] one should heat the secret wind and do the "burning spoon" [moxibustion] on secret [points for] the life-vein that makes madness.[l] This particular treatment resembles the purification of the insanity-causing demons.[m]

In general, whether [the spirits] cause insanity or cause amnesia, if due to extremely high blood and bile[n] the remedy does not take [effect], then we should substitute purification. After that, one should [give] moxibustion,[o] essences [like vitamins], the stimulant medicines [long pepper, cubeb and cardamon], and nourishing food.

To change most of the demons that cause insanity and oblivion,[p] rely upon confessions, ablutions, offering cakes, imposing truth, and peaceful ritual action. Cure the spirits seductively by water offerings, naga rituals and offering cakes.[q]

Finally, use the ultimately wrathful ritual action.[r]

Thus he spoke.

[Here ends] the seventy-ninth chapter on curing the diseases which cause amnesia, from the tantra of profound secret instruction, the eight branched essential nectar.

Chapter 79—Notes

a. Mind is rather "pushed in," "heavy," "like somebody tied it up."
b. All joints ache.
c. This describes the general character of oblivion madness, a diminishing of clarity and concentration which becomes complete oblivion and loss of memory in its chronic stages.

d.   Acts startled, jumpy; knees are stiff and rigid.

e.   Especially with bile, the illness gets worse in relationship to digestion. One hour after eating the symptoms of the disease become more intense. The path of the fire element is bile, so because digestion involves the production of heat, the bile is overstimulated. This is even more marked if the food itself is hot.

f.   Symptoms of poison are not clear from urine and pulse analysis and the doctor has difficulty in diagnosis. The effects of poison in this case is that mind is steeped in illusion—one hears and sees what is not there.

g.   As characteristic of the action of demons, all behavior in the person possessed is reversed. For example, if the person didn't drink liquor before, he will when he becomes possessed.

h.   These are preliminary purification medicines.

i.   If one uses new (fresh) liquid from inside the gall bladder of a yellow cow, one strains it and puts it up the nose to remove pus, etc. If one uses old and dried gall bladder or bile, then it needs to be mixed with water, then strained and put up the nose.

j.   A person with "the demon who causes forgetfulness" falls down a lot; sometimes he may be unconscious for up to twenty or thirty minutes. In that case, the finger tips and toe tips must be touched with a hot (burning) iron knife. The best kind of knife is one that killed nine people; the least good kind (but still usable) is one that killed one person.

k.   Barley beer and molasses—the description of how to make this medicine is in the Fourth Tantra.

l.   Top of the head, below sternum, and the Tibetan 1st, 8th and 20th vertebrae. If a person is too fat to find his vertebrae, then one uses one's thumb as a measure and counts down from the base of the neck. Here the points correspond to the seventh cervical, sixth thoracic and third sacral.

m.   Regarding moxa points.

n.   Whoever gets the madness and oblivion causing ghosts are often similar in that they have high blood and bile.

o.   Top of head and beneath sternum.

p.   That is, demons rather than organic or psychological causes.

q.   *Shi-wa*. Peaceful religious action: prayers to the Triple Gem; sadhanas of peaceful deities. These actions must be performed by a monastic lama with high realization. Also, peaceful exorcism.

Gently asking the spirits to go and seductive methods of exorcism (see exorcism section) such as putting torma in shape of person and throwing it outside.

r. "Tro-wa" (*khro-wa*). Wrathful religious rituals, sadhanas of the wrathful deities, and threatening methods of exorcism. This includes burning fires and putting the names of the ghosts in the fires (to get rid of them), or burying the names of the ghosts or objects to which the ghosts have been attracted. These wrathful acts should be performed by yogis and married lamas with high realization.

A Few Parallels to Modern Psychiatry

First of all, from the point of view of general description, the type of insanity described in Chapter 77 as the effect of elemental spirits—the sudden onset of behavior of a consistently alien nature with little physical disturbance and no perceptible organic causes—corresponds to what the Western model, which is for the most part also descriptive, classifies as functional psychosis. Particularly, the symptomatic effects of the various elemental spirits suggest schizophrenia and manic depressive psychosis.

For example, mentally ill people exhibiting the demonic effect of the gods speak religious languages in a non-violent manner and are obsessed with cleanliness, while those exhibiting the demonic effects of the pervasive spirit shout for God, fixate on religious books and rituals, are aggressive and abusive and even harm themselves, presumably in expiation for their sins. The latter correspond to *DSM* II classification 295.3: "schizophrenia, paranoid type" which exhibits "persecutory or grandiose delusions, often associated with hallucinations. Excessive religiosity is sometimes seen. The patient's attitude is frequently hostile and aggressive."[36] The former is evidence of inappropriate religious behavior often noticed in schizophrenia and other psychoses; the last four categories of ghosts in Chapter 77 are also related to this type of behavior.

Furthermore, the hebephrenic type of schizophrenia (*DSM* II type 295.1) often shows "unpredictable giggling, silly and regressive behavior and mannerisms..." like people "possessed" by scent-eater demons who like to "sing, dance, and play."[37]

The demonic effect of the anti-gods is that people "look indirectly out of the corners of their eyes...speak much reckless talk...have great pride and fierce anger," which is a nearly classic description of mania. Similarly, those exhibiting the psychotic effect of the flesh-eaters are typically depressive: they "are ashamed of themselves, have low voices and a downcast manner...faint without reason and talk disjointedly...[and] scratch at the earth and fields."

Such similar descriptions of psychopathology from the millennia old Tibetan system and modern Western psychiatry would seem to support Jung's contention that the psychopathology of schizophrenia demonstrates beyond a doubt the production of archaic motifs and structural patterns from within the unconscious.

Moreover, concerning the demons of Chapter 77 and the psychotic effects of ghosts in general, it should be noted that schizophrenics themselves often believe that they are being controlled by someone else or some outer force, and in this regard they say they have trouble distinguishing whether their thoughts are their own or the alien being's. This phenomenon fits quite naturally with the idea of possession seen in Tibetan psychiatry.

There are many other parallels one could draw in relation to the demons causing mental illness. Suffice it to add here that in Tibetan psychiatry, particularly in this millennium old text, the effects of these beings are also related to organic pathology and psychosomatic disorders. The demons of Chapter 79 express themselves in relation to physical symptoms much in the same way that psychophysiologic disorders (DSM-305) are elaborated in terms of specific physiological problems of the skin, cardiovascular, and gastrointestinal systems, etc.

Further, the effects of nutritional defects and poison stand alone as causes of psychopathology in addition to being contributing factors of becoming "possessed" by the range of unseen psycho-disturbers. Again, the DSM lists classification of psychosis with metabolic or nutritional disorders (294.1) and with poison (294.3). Treatment of the former in the Tibetan system is reminiscent of megavitamin and nutritional therapy.

Generally, the symptoms described in Chapter 78 and 79 are less marked and alien than those of 77. In Chapters 78 and 79 it is clear that Tibetan psychiatry recognizes a large number of different causes—emotional reactions, organic diseases, metabolic or humoral disturbances, nutritional disorders, and poisons as well as the lack of an apparent cause (the ghost operating by itself)—that produce similar groups of symptoms, specifically psychoneuroses (especially Chapter 78) and organic psychoses (especially Chapter 79). This compares very well to modern medical classifications of these groups, where, for example, toxic confusional states, organic dementia, thyroid "madness" and lack of an apparent cause can all come under the heading of organic psychosis. The description of symptoms in 79 is particularly reminiscent of organic dementia, in which loss of memory is one of the primary features.

These chapters also refer to the personality types and psychiatric disturbances related to the three humors, which have already been described at length; catatonia, for example, parallels the type of madness related to phlegm. The Tibetan humoral character models also parallel W.H. Sheldon's attempts to correlate body types with personality: his thin "ectomorphs" are like the Tibetan wind-types and are thought most prone to schizophrenia, the fat "endomorphs" are like the phlegm types, and the athletic "mesomorphs" are like the bile types.

Tibetan psychiatry is quite sophisticated; the logic evinced in this ancient clinical text, where three major categories of mental illness are distingiushed and defined by primary causes and secondary conditions, classes, symptoms and cures, is remarkable.

11

The Pharmacology of
Tibetan Medical Psychiatry

Additional Psychiatric Medicines

Although the *Gyu-zhi* is an ancient text, its herbal treatments are still
used today among Tibetan doctors. This is true of the whole range of
its remedies, not only its psychiatric cures.

Contemporary Tibetan doctors also use psychiatric medicines
that are not found in the psychiatric chapters of the *Gyu-zhi* we have
reviewed here. In order to fill out the picture of Tibetan psychiatric
herbal cures, I have included the recipes for five other psychiatric
medicines presently in use. All together they show a vital continuation
and elaboration of the Tibetan medical tradition of psycho-
pharmacology. Tibetan psychiatric remedies, as already noted, are
held in wide esteem by the Tibetans for their effectiveness. And to my
knowledge none of them have been analyzed or tested scientifically
for their active properties.

The first of these additional remedies is a medicine called "The
Precious Essence that Removes the Mind of Sorrow" (*Sems-kyi gdung-
sel rin-chen snying-po shes*). It is a formula described in a short medical
text attributed to the Turquoise Physician Yuthog, the famous eighth
century Tibetan physician-saint. According to the colophon of the
text, Yuthog considered this such a supreme medicine that he always
kept some of it "tucked in his collar." The text was explicated to me
by the contemporary Tibetan doctor Amchi Lama Wangla of Ghoom,
Darjeeling, a master of this particular medicine.[38]

This is a kind of spiritual super-medicine. Besides being effective against mental illness and various associated physical complaints, it can be taken in small doses (one pill a day) as a super-strengthening tonic.

When asked which, if any, Tibetan medicine would be helpful for the mental illness so widespread in the modern world, H.H. Dudjom Rinpoche answered this "Precious Essence." The text for this psychiatric remedy, which has been continuously used and held in high regard for over a thousand years, reads as follows:

OM SWASTI! This is called "The Precious Essence that Removes the Mind of Sorrow," a written medicine which is kept extremely secret.

Collect together *Costus speciosus,* sweet flag rhizome, long pepper, wild ginger, black salt, and, in a weight equal to those, golden skinned myrobalan [here Lama Wangla also added black aloeswood]. Again, equal to all that "the yak of the supreme medicine" [a synonym for the best kind of black aconite]. Then add as much nutmeg as equals all of that.

Over that, precious detoxified mercury.[39] [Now, how to detoxify it, with:] A dram of pure sulphur [*mu-se*] mixed with a dram of mercury; keep grinding it for half a day. In addition, put together with it as much as you can get of many kinds of hearts—the blood of a healthy parrot and the heart of a wild northern yak, etc. Especially, add to that other powerful medicines if you know them. Anyhow, grind all those together into a very find powder. During the three days [of purifying mercury] add the urine of an eight year old child so it is absorbed [keeping the mixture the consistency of mud].

When it becomes an indigo color, [having combined it with the other ingredients] make it into pills about the size of a pea. Bless it in a precious vessel with mendrup and by repeating the auspicious mantra [of Sanskrit vowels and consonants] at exactly just past noon.

By giving 3, 5, or 7 pills, as necessary, there is nothing that cannot be subdued by this method; especially all heart-wind diseases [*snying-rlung nad*—including emotional illness of both violent and depressive types, stress disorders, high blood pressure, and heart disease], insane crying and shouting, serious loss of sensibility, hiccups, a mind that grows fearful and sad without reason, big wild anger, forgetting everything, foggy vision, and pain in the upper chest when filling up with breath.

Especially for diseases that are very difficult to treat and for those generated by evil forces, this medicine is supreme even by just having it in the house [—which can prevent these types of karmic disease].

Also, other diseases—of phlegm, bile and lymph, cold and worms [microorganisms]; in fact, all hot and cold diseases caused by the three humors are subdued by this supreme medicine, which Yuthog always kept tucked in a little bag inside his collar.

This is the wealth of the father of skilled doctors [Yuthog] of Trong-tse. EMAHO! Wonderful!

The next medicine is an all-purpose psychiatric incense made and used by Dodrag Amchi, a lama-doctor in Bodhnath, Nepal. According to him, this incense is good for all types of mental disturbances, insanity and emotional instability. A pinch of it is burned on a coal; the patient puts his head over it, a cloth on his head draping over it like a tent from inside of which he inhales all the smoke. The incense mixture contains ground:

> black aloeswood exudate
> frankincense from the white-grey aloeswood
> frankincense from the red aloeswood
> white frankincense from the Sal tree
> black frankincense from the Indian bedellium
> nutmeg
> cubeb
> juniper
> chebulic myrobalan
> beleric myrobalan
> emblic myrobalan
> *Delfinium grandflorium.*

The next three psychiatric remedies[40] come from a little booklet called *The Gist Prescriptions of Tibetan Traditional Medicines.* This booklet is published by the Tibetan Medical Centre in Dharamsala, India, and lists one hundred and fifty medicines that are available today through the Medical Centre and used primarily by the Tibetan refugee community there. The first seventeen medicines listed are for stress and emotional problems. Some of these are exactly the same as remedies described in the Second Tantra of the *Gyu-zhi.*

The text of the booklet is in Tibetan. It describes the disorder and says how to take the medicine, but it does not list the ingredients. The Tibetan names of the ingredients were kindly supplied by the Director of the Medical Centre.

Gist remedy number one is called "Asafoetida Plus Twenty-Five." It is described as follows: "Take a dose of this medicine at dawn or dusk, whichever is convenient, to benefit diseases of wind in the upper, lower and mid-parts of the body caused by the outer wind entering the pores of the skin, the flesh and the veins, the inner wind entering the five solid organs such as the heart, etc. and the six hollow organs such as the stomach, etc., and the secret wind entering the life force and the psychic channels."

It contains:

> asafoetida
> nutmeg
> black aloeswood
> the "Six Good Things": cloves, saffron, true cardamon, cubeb, bamboo pith, and nutmeg
> black frankincense from Indian bedellium
> white frankincense from the Sal tree
> elecampane
> *Adhatoda vasica*
> blue lotus
> bamboo pith

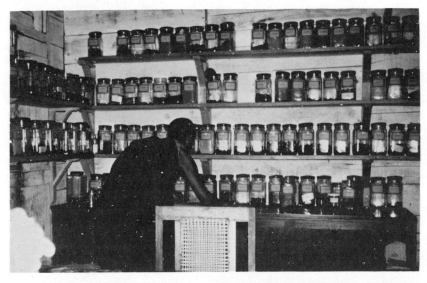

Figure 37 The dispensary at the Tibetan Medical Centre in Dharamsala. On the shelves are some of the hundreds of medicine pills, powders, etc., made and prescribed according to traditional formulae. Many of these medicines, including psychiatric medications, have been in continuous use among Tibetans for over a thousand years.

chebulic myrobalan
clove
nying-sho
"human flesh"
the "Three Hots": ginger, long pepper, black pepper
various hearts.

Another medicine is *Gist #12,* which is entitled "Eleven Life Sustainers." The text says, "Take this medicine with tepid boiled water in the morning or evening, whichever is convenient, when there is pain in the upper chest, upper back, breasts and diaphragm, when speech is mute, and when mental consciousness is disturbed because agitated wind has entered the heart center and life vein."

It contains:

black aloeswood
nutmeg
nying-sho
bamboo pith
white frankincense from the Sal tree
Costus speciosus
chebulic myrobalan
cobra's saffron
clove
"human flesh"
asafoetida.

Finally, there is *Gist #13:* "Mental Happiness." The text says, "Take one dose of this medicine in the morning or evening, whichever is convenient, with beer, bone soup or boiled water for diseases arising from wind and especially mental depression, often accompanied with trembling, caused by the wind entering into the life vein so that consciousness no longer dwells in its natural place."

It contains:

mercury
black aloeswood
clove
nutmeg
aconite
the "Three Hots": ginger, long pepper, black pepper
heart of a rabbit
heart of a wild yak
heart of a dri
various hearts.

Important Tibetan Psychopharmacology and Problems of Identification

The problems involved in identifying Tibetan pharmacological substances are numerous. Tibetans never had a systematic classification for plants like we have in the West, and so there is a great deal of difficulty in identifying Tibetan materia medica as a result. Major medicinal substances had different names in different parts of Tibet, and even these changed over the centuries. Furthermore, different substances have the same name in different locations in Tibet.

Most medicinal substances from the animal, mineral, and vegetable worlds had many different synonyms even within one region of Tibet. Myrobalan (Tib. *a-ru-ra*), for example, has at least thirty-seven synonyms in Tibetan and forty-two in Sanskrit. What is more, while animal substances are frequently used in medicines, medicines bearing animal names can be misleading for they may not refer to an animal part at all but may be the synonym for a medicine plant. Theodore Burang illustrated this problem:

> In identifying Tibetan materia medica one can easily slip up and make serious mistakes. For example: *ne-zen* is a substance sometimes used for healing purposes. In Western translation it was rendered as 'sparrow's flesh.' What it really means though is barley-corn which has been eaten by sparrows and partially processed in the digestive tract, then removed from the entrails of recently dead sparrows and used as an admixture in medicinal compounds.[41]

In addition, much of the medical teaching is based on oral transmission, and without the oral transmission the real meaning of the written names of the substances can not be known. The information was meant to be secret, the real meaning being imparted only to the most worthy students.

Since, unfortunately, most Tibetan lamas and doctors, even those few who speak English, are not well versed in Western botanical (or medical) terms, it will take a joint effort by Western botanists and Tibetan doctors to produce the identification of the most important substances used in Tibetan medicine. Such an effort would be a great contribution to the scientific study of Tibetan medicine, but to date the work has not been done. And without such a basis to go on, the business of translating the names of the materia medica is risky at best.

Perhaps it is because of this that although there are many herbals and works on pharmacology in Tibetan, there has been no translation of any of them into English with the corresponding Latin terminology. The Chinese, I have heard, have produced a book in Tibet that lists Tibetan pharmacology and gives their Chinese botanical equivalents. However, I was never able to find a copy of this book either in India or in the West.

Therefore, in order to identify the Tibetan pharmacology in the texts I have presented in this work, I have had to rely on a variety of reference works in English, and these do not necessarily agree on the meaning of the pharmacological terms or even list them at all.

The best reference work in English that includes the subject is the Chandra Das *Tibetan English Dictionary,* published in 1902—hardly a modern work yet still very excellent. It does not, however, include all pharmacological ingredients and in many cases does not give the Latin or English names, just identifying things as medicinal substances.

One of the most useful features of the Chandra Das is that it gives quotes from Tibetan medical works on the properties of the various substances, and these additional descriptions are very informative. Also helpful for identification is Jäschke's Tibetan-English dictionary, but it is even earlier than the Chandra Das. Dhongthog's modern English-Tibetan dictionary is helpful for verifying the names of common substances.

There is a work in Russian which cross-references the Tibetan, Latin, and Russian names. Again, not all ingredients are included and there are a few problems with inaccuracies. Still, it is a comprehensive work and the best available (Gammerman).

Also helpful is an unpublished Tibetan-Sanskrit work by Professor Dr. Lokesh Chandra which lists the corresponding terms from an ancient Sanskrit Ayurvedic work and its Tibetan equivalents.

Major works on medicinal substances of the Orient, like those of Chopra, Dastur, Jain, etc., have also been referred to.

On the basis of the above cited works, I have been able to make a tentative identification of the substances named in the psychiatric medicines and texts presented in this book. This material is found in the charts of Tibetan psycho-pharmacology in the appendix. These charts were reviewed and corrected at an early stage by the Indian Ayurvedic scholar and physician, Dr. Vaidya Bhagwan Dash.

From the research found in these charts, we can enumerate some of the main substances used in Tibetan medicine for treating mental illness. These are aconite, asafoetida, *Costus speciosus,* nutmeg, clove, sweet flag and varieties of frankincense and incense.

Aconite, *Aconitum (bong-nga).* Aconite is such a great poison that even in handling it one is in danger and must be careful not to inhale its dust, which can destroy the mucus lining of the throat and stomach. It is important that it be used with certain other ingredients which nullify its toxicity.

There are seven main varieties of aconite that grow in the Himalayas, and all of these vary in quality and effect depending on where they are grown. Medicine recipes usually call for one type or another. Black aconite is the strongest and most powerful species. One of its synonyms is "Great Medicine." Only small amounts are used.

Aconite is known in modern herbal pharmacology as a sedative and depressant. According to Tibetans, it cures heart diseases caused by excess of air—not just physical heart disease but disturbances of the heart-center that lead to mental imbalance and distortion. It was once much used in the West in cardiac and respiratory therapy.

Asafoetida, *Ferula assafoetida (shing-kun).* The part used is the exudate from the root of the plant. It is known in modern herbalism as a stimulant to the brain and nervous system as well as a sedative, expectorant, tonic, laxative, diuretic and aphrodisiac. According to the Tibetans, it cures disturbances of air at the heart center, impotency and degeneration of the organism caused by aging.

Medicines are often graded by the Tibetans as "best," "middle," and "least." Dr. Ama Lobsang, the well-known Tibetan woman doctor in Dharamsala, called asafoetida the "best" among psychiatric materia medica. She said that after it is cleaned and made into a boiled concoction and mixed with milk, it works as a powerful medicine and sleeping potion. The quality of asafoetida is tested by cutting the stem and drawing a white string across it twice. If the string turns blue, it is of superior quality.

Ru-rta, *Costus speciosus.** This is a light brown spicy root that predominates in Tibetan psychiatric prescriptions. The root is similar to that of the plant *ma-nu (Inula helenium* or elecampane), which is also

---

*Ru-rta may also be *Saussurea lappa* or costusroot, as it is called in English. The two entirely different plants—*Costus speciosus* and *Saussurea lappa*—have been much confused and hence misidentified with each other in scientific literature.

called *ma-nu ru-rta* and was formerly used in Western medicine as a remedy for pulmonary diseases.

According to the Tibetans, the root known as *ru-rta* regulates blood pressure and the wind at the heart; it also expels afterbirth, relieves suppressed menses and abdominal distension, and is useful in pulmonary disorders.

Nutmeg, *Myristica fragans* (*dzaa-ti*). Nutmeg is specifically used for all disturbances of the winds, especially the life-wind, and the heart center. In fact, if no other medicine is available for psychiatric problems, then it is said that nutmeg, "King of Incenses," can be used alone as an effective cure through inhalation. It is sometimes used in the West for its psychedelic effects, but can be toxic if used incorrectly.

Clove, *Caryophyllus aromaticus* (*li-shi*). Clove is specifically for the *srog-rtsa,* the life-vein or vital channel (probably the vagus) which is connected to the heart and where the subtle life-force serving as a mount for consciousness resides. It is also good for the subtle veins of consciousness at the heart center.

Clove is used for most all types of wind disorders of a psychiatric nature, also for cardiac wind disorders, including angina pectoris. Clove's power is warming; it generates body heat and is good for digestion.

Sweet flag, *Acorus calamus* (*shu-dag*). The aromatic rhizome is the part used in medicine. Among its many properties, it is known in Western herbalism as a sedative excellent for insomnia and nervousness.

Frankincense and Aromatics. The Tibetans distinguished many kinds of frankincenses and aromatic substances excellent for use in psychiatric incenses. They are held to be especially sacred. Among them, black aloeswood, *Aquilara agallocha* (*a-ga-ru*), can even be used alone for particular psychiatric cases involving "demonic spirits." The black and white kinds of frankincenses obtained from the Indian bedellium, *Commiphora mukul* (*gu-gul*), "the ghost's fear," and from the Sal tree, *Shorea robusta* (*spos-dkar*), are also in this category. The berries of the Himalayan Juniper, *Juniperius psendosabina* (*shug-pa*), are similarly burned as incense to counter delerium. Most of these ingredients are used in oral medicines and medicinal ointments as well as in incenses.

Of these, it is black aloeswood which contemporary Tibetan doctors primarily rely upon for the treatment of the whole range of nervous and emotional disorders—anxiety, depression, excitability, etc.—that comes under the heading "lung," disturbances of the life-wind at the heart center. Black aloeswood is the most commonly used minor tranquilizer. Other ingredients that are regularly compounded in psychiatric medications are long pepper, cardamon, cubeb and pine.

It is important to remember of these and other ingredients in the psychiatric remedies that it is their combination, the way they work with each other, that is the synergy that empowers the transformation or cure. So we can't know, without scientific investigation that does not exclude all the subtle components and considerations, if one or two or all ingredients work together to give the healing effect or if some of the ingredients are included simply as a matter of tradition. It will certainly be worth investigating, however.

We should remember that *Rauwolfia serpentina* was a well known Indian Ayurvedic cure for insanity. In the mid-20th century it was given serious scientific attention and, scientists having isolated the active alkaloids from the root of the plant, *Rauwolfia serpentina* spawned a large number of anti-psychotic drugs (reserpine—Sandril, Serpasil; Moderil; Harmonyl). In short, the old Ayurvedic cure, when examined, ushered in a whole new era of psychiatric treatment: psychopharmacology—medications under the heading of "the organic approach." The very old became the very new and revolutionized the care and treatment of the insane.

In order to appreciate the significance of this contribution one only has to remember that just prior to it mentally ill people were kept in padded cells and straight-jackets—and prior to that, for centuries and centuries (and even as recently as one hundred years ago) they were kept in chains and cages and were treated or,. more correctly, abused in the most gruesome and barbaric manner.

Of course, in some sense modern psychiatric drugs can be said to have removed the iron chains from the body and replaced them with chemical chains on the mind. And certainly, as is widely agreed, these tranquilizing drugs are very imperfect, have dangerous side-effects and are tremendously over-prescribed. Nevertheless, they represent a major advancement in psychiatric medicine; and, hopefully, better, more effective and less dangerous medications will be discovered in the future.

In general, Tibetan doctors do not think it advisable to use the strongest medicines first. This is because they do not wish to displace symptoms but, rather, to get to the root cause instead. Also, they use restraint because the strongest medicinal substances may have adverse effects. For example, asafoetida medicine butter (eaten or applied to the skin) is said to be extremely effective against psychosis. But a Tibetan text advises that in the cases of very intelligent people who have become psychotic, it is better to treat them with less strong medicines first so as not to impair their intellectual capacities. In some cases, of course, it may still be necessary to use the stronger medicines.

As for the inclusion of substances such as blood and urine in medicines, it may strike the modern mind as disgusting and outrageous. But such substances are found in traditional medicines around the world, including China, and sometimes turn out, under scientific investigation, to have some merit. Urine, for example, has recently been found to contain substances that act as powerful mental and emotional tranquilizers without any of the side-effects of manufactured chemical tranquilizers—according to Danish scientists.

Most Tibetan psychiatric medicines, even those including the strongest substances, are slow working, harmless, and long lasting. They are not meant to have a radical and disruptive effect on the system.

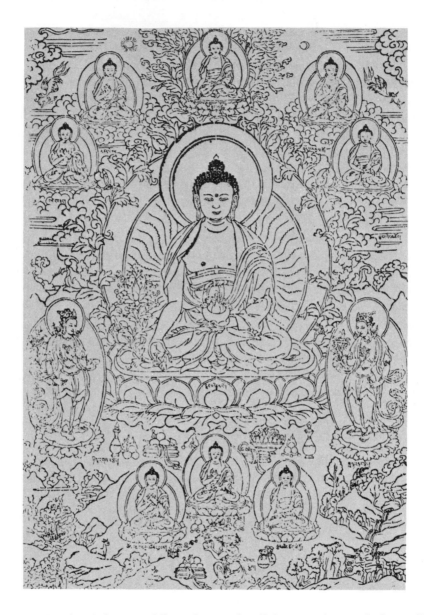

Figure 38 The Medicine Buddha in his paradise "Pleasing When Looked Upon" with Shakyamuni Buddha above his head and surrounded by the seven manifestations of Healing Buddhas. He is attended by two medicine goddesses "Like the Sun" and "Like the Moon" who dispel all the diseases of cold or heat. This medicine paradise is a place beyond ordinary perception, a place within the perfection of wisdom.

12

Concluding Remarks and Flights of Thought

The preceding pages have been an attempt to present the ancient system of Tibetan Buddhist medicine and psychiatry in its religious, philosophical, cultural and medical contexts.

We have seen that the beginning of this medical system was with the second millennium B.C. in Vedic India; that the Buddha himself spoke of truth in its terms; that the development of Buddhism polished it; and that at the time of its greatest radiance in India the jewel of Indian Buddhism and Ayurveda was protected from destruction and enshrined in the highest land on earth to flourish there up until our own times. And now the forces of time and history and materialism theaten to bury this healing jewel, the diamond healing, one of the oldest continuous systems of medicine in the world and one of immense ethical, philosophical and spiritual depth.

That all forms die sooner or later is the inevitable course of impermanence and the cause of suffering which Buddhist medicine cures. But as the Medicine Buddha is innate in the Primordial Buddha, so may the inspiration and insight of Tibetan medicine find new expressions in yet unimagined ways.

On the surface, perhaps, especially to someone unfamiliar with the terms of Tibetan Buddhist medicine, it seems remote and alien, especially Tibetan psychiatry. But we have looked below the surface and have found its philosophical and religious foundations are those which concern the nature of mind and consciousness. The Buddhist language which expresses these concepts may be a foreign tongue, but we still share the experience.

Especially are the voices which tell of madness very different in the Tibetan culture from those in our own. Their ghosts are our psychoses; their subtle consciousness veins where the "mind rides the winds" are our neural synapses and biochemical interactions.

The parallels between specific types of psychopathology in the Tibetan traditions and modern psychiatry have already been noted in previous chapters. But there are many other points of meeting and comparison between the ancient Tibetan and the modern Western psychiatric traditions.

Freud insisted that one could not treat and cure psychiatric disorders without first understanding the nature of the disease. Proceeding from that standpoint, he brought psychology into the realm of the natural sciences and clinical observation. This the Tibetans never did in the modern sense, but they had, in their own terms and language, a way of understanding the nature and source of illness based on Buddhist psychology, a rational system of classifying mental illness according to observable symptoms and etiology, and a wide range of treatments to cure it.

The whole psychosomatic approach to healing in Tibetan medicine is instructive. Since mind is understood to be the source of both illness and wellness, Tibetan medicine integrates mental, spiritual and mystical healing techniques with the practice of regular medicine. Various meditative and ritual practices heal on an internal plane and are designed to integrate, purify and transform the psyche.

In psychiatric treatment, the whole range of practices is integrated so that neither the psychological approach, the physiological approach, nor the environmental approach is dwelled on exclusively, but rather they are used together as a holistic treatment model. Thus, the wide range of unique, complex and sophisticated natural medicines, as well as medical treatments like acupuncture and specialized massage and exercise, are combined with a program of specific alterations of lifestyle, behavior, diet, etc., as well as spiritual medications and meditations to catalyze the self-curative powers of mind and body.

In fact, a whole premise of modern milieu therapy and the therapeutic community is prefigured in the Tibetan system. Diet is elaborated in terms of its effects and healing power. The color, temperature, and type of environment which best promote recovery are delineated in terms of the humoral types. The importance of the state of mind of nurses, doctors, therapists and friends in attendance is specifically emphasized.

This type of treatment is basically a kind of naturopathy which was utilized by the classical Romans and Greeks in their treatment of insanity, an essentially humane and rational approach. Unfortunately for the mad folks who lived between then and the 20th century in the West, that kind of treatment was mostly abandoned until this century.

We can say that the importance which Tibetan Buddhist psychiatry assigns to the high development of morality and kindness on the healer's part has not been without adherents in the West, but it is not, in general, held to be a critical aspect of the healing process and has never been developed systematically as it was in the Tibetan system through the figure of the Medicine Buddha.

Modern medical commentators have stated that in order for there to be a psychiatric cure it is important that there be faith in the therapist, and the Tibetans would certainly agree. They understood the self-curative power of mind and they designed practices to activate it. Further, their model of the healer is the highest possible: the Medicine Buddha. The actual healer who aspires to that level and develops his skill, wisdom, and compassion accordingly is worthy of faith and can engender it in others.

Considering its antiquity, Tibetan psychiatry is remarkably sophisticated from the psychological point of view. In a simple but basic way it takes into account the psychological causes of mental illness both operating by themselves and in conjunction with biological, behavioral, environmental, and spiritual factors.

The description of the effect of demonic forces causing mental illness that we have detailed comes from a medical text that is approximately one thousand years old. Modern Tibetan doctors do not speak of demons and ghosts in the archaic way, but rather as invisible energies and forces that can and do affect consciousness. They may be understood to come from within—the unconscious, our "other selves," and the collective unconscious, and from without— from other people, places, or planets.

Invisible negative forces, of course, are only one cause of mental illness, according to the Tibetans. The other causes are organic and psychological. But even in discussing madness caused by possession by demonic forces, the tradition mentions the precipitating psychological factors. We should remember that an understanding of psychological causes and motivation related to insanity did not emerge in Western psychology until the 18th century.

For example, some of the causes of unseen negative forces taking hold of a person and making him mad—and these are also understood to be causes of madness by themselves—are isolation, breaking vows and promises, "sinning," loss of possessions or loved ones or self-esteem, and fixation on emotional pain. Regarding the latter, we can compare it to what Norbert Wiener called the "cybernetic machine" in which a "vicious cycle of morbid ideas" takes hold of and intensifies the melancholic personality. Egas Moniz also observed a similar process:

> ...obsessive and melancholic—have a circumscribed mental existence confined to a limited cycle of ideas which, dominating all others, constantly revolved in the patient's diseased brain.[42]

Unfortunately for his patients, this led Moniz to cut out parts of the "diseased brain" with a frontal lobotomy, something no Tibetan would dream of doing not only because they disregarded the brain as an organ of consciousness, but also because they would never hold such an isolated, specialized view of psychophysical processes or attack and treat symptoms in such a radical way while disregarding the deeper causes. They exercised restraint for practical if spiritual reasons—the cause would only manifest in a worse way later in future lives.

Regarding the loss of loved ones, possessions, stature, and self-esteem, these are all presently accepted stress factors, the causes of emotional instability and depression. And finally, regarding the religious causes of breaking promises and sinning, these ideas are not without parallel in the Western psychiatric tradition.

The psychiatrist Heinroth (1773-1843) held that the ultimate cause of mental disturbances was "sin." And what he meant by that was very close to what the Buddhists mean: selfishness, the instinctual and intellectual self-aggrandizing ego. What is more, Heinroth said that the highest level of ego-development was an assimilation of conscience, a spiritual altruism that sought the well-being of others. In short, what he described is the Mahayana Buddhist ideal: the bodhisattva.

The "sin" which Heinroth referred to is called "sense of guilt" in modern psychiatry. It results from "inner conflict," from offending one's moral sense, and it produces mental disturbances.

In modern psychoanalysis as described by Freud, the analyst works to free the energy which is bound up in inner conflict and to integrate the unconscious with the ego, superego, and the demands of reality. Buddhist psychology agrees with this goal but, in the direction Heinroth indicated, goes beyond integrating the unconscious, the ego, and the superego to bring about a level of integration than can freely and readily seek the well-being of others.

The Buddhist idea is to transform unconscious motivation and inner conflict, having understood it, into conscious bodhisattva intention: to generate the thought of enlightenment for all beings and to act in their behalf. This is the Buddhist compassion which must always be exercised in conjunction with wisdom (and vice versa) and which arises spontaneously with it. In this compassion there can be no smug self-satisfaction with petty acts of kindness, for it is the motivation (whether for self or for others) that renders an action compassionate or selfish.

The bodhisattva path is an open, non-defensive, non-judgmental way of being, of loving. And by definition it entails a constant openness to critical self-evaluation as the way to truth and freedom. In this it is similar to psychoanalysis. As Erich Fromm put it, "Both in humanistic religious thinking and in psychoanalysis man's ability to search for truth is held to be inseparably linked to the attainment of freedom and independence."[43]

This bring us back to religion and to the basic Buddhist philosophical and psychological orientation that is so integral a part of Tibetan medicine and psychiatry. In founding what was to become one of the world's major religions, and its only major psychological religion, the Buddha, it can be claimed, became the world's first great introspective psychologist. His entire philosophy, and the medical system which adjoins it, is based on an analysis of mind. Through fearless introspection, not reliance on God or supernatural aids, did the Prince Gautama become the Buddha. As such, he is a model of human perfection. His doctrine, the Dharma, is not a rigid theology but a support (one of the literal meanings of the word "dharma") for the search for the real meaning in life and for the attempt to comprehend oneself, one's mind and the nature of one's experience.

The entire thrust of the Buddha's teaching and the Buddha's path is to encounter the mind, become aware of how it works and how it controls us, and then to bring it under control and through this to cure suffering. For according to Buddhism, the source of all physical and mental disease and suffering is the lack of control of mind.

The Dharma has the ultimate goal of alleviating suffering, not just the suffering of the sick and miserable as opposed to the healthy and fortunate, but the suffering and neuroses we all share by virtue of our egotism, ignorance, lusts and hates. There is a Buddhist axiom in the Pali tradition: *Subbe putha jana ummattaka,* "All worldlings are deranged." As one writer has commented, this "indicates the whole purpose of Buddhism is to apply mental therapy to a condition which, accepted as the norm, is in truth nothing but a universal delusion."[44]

In attempting to heal the derangement of worldlings, the Buddha can be said to have developed a form of psychotherapy, and in fact numerous writers have remarked upon this aspect of Buddhism. Conversely, modern psychologists like Erich Fromm have perceived a basically religious function in psychoanalysis, which Fromm describes as a "cure for the soul."

The means of mental therapy employed by the Buddha, the "Great Physician" and great psychologist, are not, of course, psychoanalysis but a transformation of self through the development of morality, meditation, and wisdom. Through meditation in particular one can become aware of unconscious motivations, mental habits and inner conflicts, and free oneself of bondage to them.

In the process of meditation, the repressive strictures of the "superego" are consciously relaxed so that all kinds of emotional and mental material surface. It is the process of watching the mind at work, letting the material surface without rejecting any of it, thus at the same time integrating it and breaking its hold. Unconscious motivations and unacceptable impulses are, in Buddhist terms, the inveterate propensities of defiled mind that perpetuate the cycles of existence. Meditation is a way of releasing unconscious material into consciousness so that one becomes aware of it and at the same time lessens its grip. This process is not so very different from the Freudian idea that when the origin and pattern of a personality disorder is known and brought to awareness, its influence on unconscious motivation will disappear.

However, the Buddhist model takes this further, saying that beyond the analytical "seeing" and the freedom it brings there is a "seeing" from the point of view of absolute reality—seeing that everything arises from voidness. This realization of emptiness, which can only be achieved in meditation, liberates the hold of even the most subtle and ingrained psychic patterns. Through it habits inherited from countless lifetimes begin to dissolve and from within, like a sky cleared of clouds, the light of wisdom begins to dawn.

Through meditation and the range of Buddhist practices a transformation of the personality takes place. The "ego," in the Western sense of a healthy, integrated and rationally functioning personality, is not lost but strengthened by the loss of what Eastern tradition calls "ego"—selfish, infantile craving, attachment, and anxiety. The Buddhist idea is to break out of the confines of neuroses and conditioning into a vast and open perspective beyond self and selfishness. (In this it is comparable to modern ideas of transpersonal psychology.)[45]

In his book *The Self in Transformation* Herbert Fingarette has drawn a clear parallel between basic Buddhist philosophy and psychology and Western psychoanalysis. "Persons who have failed to achieve such harmonious integration [of ego]," writes Fingarette, "meet with obstacles whose nature they do not understand (ignorance), or they are driven by 'intense defiance or greed or hostile impulses.' Ignorance, pride, lust and hatred—here is the universally acknowledged 'syndrome' associated by mystics with the disease of selfishness. The psychoanalytic explanation of neurosis is analagous. Unsublimated libido and aggression (lust, hatred and greed) result in distorted, fantasy-colored experiences ('ignorance,' 'illusion')."[46]

Through developing control of mind and powers of concentration one may achieve states of deep meditation which result eventually in realization of enlightenment. Such meditation transcends discursive mental processes. It is mystical in the sense that it transcends the duality of self and other and is a direct gnostic experience of truth and reality. But this condition of mind and being has often been misunderstood in the West. For example, medical historians and psychiatrists like Alexander and Selesnick have maintained that it is narcissistic, antisocial and regressive absorption. "Nirvana," they have written, "is a psychological and physiolgoical regression to a pre-natal state of oblivion."[47]

But, as we have seen, Tibetan Buddhist medicine considers oblivion to be a state of extreme psychopathology. Full awareness, not oblivion, is the quality of nirvana. Furthermore, as we have also discussed, the pre-natal state is described by Buddhists as being conscious and full of suffering.

The Buddha stated that the pain of being born was one of the four primary sufferings. But not only does Buddhism recognize the birth trauma, which is so important in Western psychology, it also recognizes the traumatic suffering experienced in the womb—an entirely different picture from the Western one of blissful pre-natal

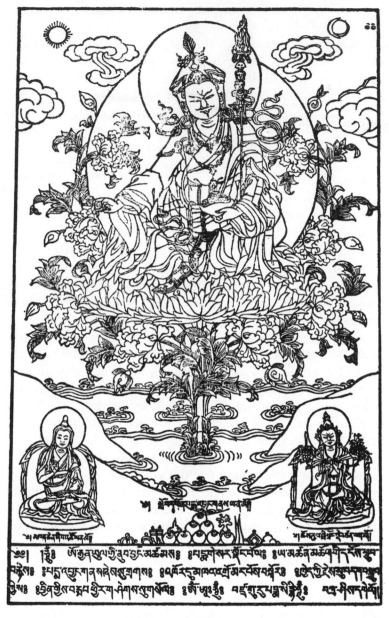

Figure 39 Guru Padmasambhava with Abbot Shantarakshita on his right and King Trison Detsen on his left. Together they established the Buddha's medicine of Dharma, the meditation practices of the healing deities, and the medical teachings of the *Gyu-zhi* in Tibet 1,200 years ago. All the teachings of Tibetan Buddhist medicine survived until the present era when sudden changes caused the culture that preserved them to all but disappear. What survives, in exile, of Tibetan medicine now encounters the modern world. Padmasambhava, the Abbot and the King all prayed these teachings would benefit beings of the future; may it prove to be so.

oblivion. Tibetan tradition delineates the range of suffering and consciousness experienced in the womb in great detail.

Freud stated that the Oedipal complex was at the core of every neurosis and that prototypical anxiety was generated by our earliest separation experiences. He managed to place sexuality and the anxiety surrounding it smack at the center of psychopathlogy.

The Tibetan tradition certainly does not disregard the importance of sexuality in mental illness. Desire, lust, and craving are the basic mental-emotional feelings that affect the inner humoral winds, and the stability of mind is directly related to the condition of the winds, particularly the life-wind. Disturbances of the life-wind are involved, either primarily or secondarily, in all psychiatric disorders. So the functioning of the libido is central to the condition of mind. In appropriate psychiatric cases sexual intercourse was prescribed as therapy. An active sexual life was culturally accepted and considered to be necessary for good health from a medical point of view. Methods for disciplining, sublimating, transcending or transforming the sex drive, on the other hand, form a part of spiritual practice. Repression in the sense that we know it is considered positively unhealthy, physically and mentally.

Tibetan Buddhist theory is remarkably "Freudian" with regard to the Oedipal complex since it fixes attraction to one parent and repulsion from the other as the cause of the karmic mind-stream of consciousness being attracted to the womb and rebirth. This is clearly stated in the *Gyu-zhi*: "It is essential that attraction to one parent and aversion to the other is felt in order that a new body should be born. If neither of these feelings takes place, there occurs no conception and no birth."[48]

However, Tibetan medicine does not expressly develop the Oedipal complex in its psychological ramifications after birth. But it is interesting that the identification with the essence of one parent ("semen" or "menstrual blood") entails hatred of that same parent and attraction to the other. This indicates a fundamental psychic division, a dualistic tendency that we are born with. Dharma practice works to reintegrate this basic split and fragmentation.

In general, it can be said that Tibetan Buddhist psychiatry is suprisingly modern in its view of the dynamic nature of psychological processes. It recognizes no permanent self-entity, just an impermanent, changing flux of reactions and perceptions, hopes and fears, habits and motivations, which we project on the external world (and in so doing, manifest it) until we recognize the dynamic process for what it is and how it arises. With that recognition we can enter the path to enlightenment.

The primacy of mind and its projections and perceptions is the center of Buddhist philosophy, psychology and psychiatry. As Padmasambhava said in *The Tibetan Book of the Great Liberation,*

> All appearances are verily one's own concepts, self-conceived in the mind, like a reflection seen in a mirror.
>
> The Dharma being nowhere save in the mind, there is no other place of meditation than the mind.
>
> Quite impossible is it to find the Buddha. . .elsewhere than the mind.[49]

Tibetan Buddhist medicine and psychiatry provides us with an inspirational and holistic model of health and healing that we in the West might benefit from contemplating. The central image of Tibetan Buddhism is also the central image of Tibetan psychiatry. It is the symbol of the ritual bell (the wisdom of blissful voidness) and the vajra-thunderbolt (the skillful means of compassion) held in two hands crossed at the heart. This is the purity and clarity of the diamond emptiness and its splendid light of manifestation brought together for the benefit of all. This is the diamond healing. It symbolically reminds us that we must blend our advanced medical technology with the life of the heart and spirit if we are to heal and be healed.

> May all of us who share a connection with
> the Buddha of Medicine be inspired
> by illumination,
> May the blessings of health and ease
> shower like fragrant blossoms from
> the Medicine Paradise,
> May the Dharma increase; may all beings
> be happy and realize the Great Perfection.

Appendix I

Charts of Substances in Tibetan Psychiatric Remedies

These charts provide a basic index of Tibetan psycho-pharmacology which may be corrected and expanded in the future. The Tibetan terms come from the Tibetan texts covered in this book. The Latin and English equivalents are the research variables. Where there is some question about the many versions of the term, I have included more than one translation.

The listings of information reflect only what the Tibetan tradition has to say about the substances, and only in a limited fashion. Occasionally a Tibetan synonym is included.

For each substance there is an indication of where the ingredient occurs in our sources. They are abbreviated as follows: Chapters 77, 78, and 79 of the Third Tantra of the *Gyu-zhi* are G-Z 77, 78, 79; The Precious Essence Which Removes the Mind of Sorrow is Prec. Ess.; the All-purpose Psychiatric Incense is Psych. Incen.; and the Gist Prescriptions are Gist 1, 12, and 13.

Altogether, these represent the ingredients used in nineteen different Tibetan psychiatric remedies—fourteen from the three chapters of the *Gyu-zhi* and five from other sources. This listing of nearly one hundred substances reflects the astonishing breadth, vitality and sophistication of psychopharmacology in Tibetan medicine, a millennial old tradition of active practice.

Tibetan Script	Tibetan Name	Latin Name	English Name	Information
གཀོལ	Ka-ko-la	Piper cubeba or Amomun sabulatum	Cubeb Greater Cardamon	One of the "Six Good Things." Good for the spleen. G-Z 78—thrice, 79. Psych. Incen., Gist 1.
སྐྱུརུར	sKyu-ru-ra	Emblica officinalis	Emblic myrobalan	Sour fruit said to cure diseases of phlegm and air. Increases bile. One of the "Three Chief Fruits." G-Z 77, 78—twice. Psych. Incen.
སྐྱེརཔ	sKyer-pa	Berberis aristata	Indian barberry	Flower to cure diarrhea; fruit to draw out bilious matter; bark useful in dropsy. Very cooling. G-Z 77.
ཁརུཚ	Kha-ru-tsha		A black salt (made with myrobalan, fused together in boiling producing a nitrate of soda)	One of three precious substances keeping in the life-wind. Overcomes flatulence, phlegm and wind. G-Z 78, Prec. Ess.
གནྡྷཔད	Gandha-pa-tra	Fanacetum sibiricum		A fragrant herb with yellow flower. G-Z 77.
གུགུལ	Gu-gul	Commiphora mukul	Indian bedellium	Frankincense. The oleo-gum-resin. The sacred black variety of the resinous exudate. Its smell is said to drive away evil spirits. Tib. syn.: "the ghost's fear." Psych. Incen., Gist 1.

Tibetan Script	Tibetan Name	Latin Name	English Name	Information
གུར་གུམ།	Gur-gum	Crocus sativus	Saffron crocus	Cures all diseases of heat. Good for liver. Good against bile disorders. In Chinese herbal literature it is called "Tibetan safflower." G-Z 77, 78—twice. Gist 1.
རྒྱ་སྤོས། རྒྱམ་ཚྭ།	rGya-spos rGyam-tshwa	Valeriana wallichi	Indian valerian Sea salt	G-Z 77, 78 G-Z 78.
སྒེ་གསེར།	sGe-gsher	Zingiber officinale	Ginger	Ginger removes phlegm and wind and liquifies the blood. G-Z 78.
སྒྲོན་ཤིང།	sGron-shing	Pinus silvestris Pinus picea	Pine	Removes mucus, cold, and wind in the stomach. G-Z 77—twice, 78—twice. Gist 1, 13.
དངུལ་ཆུ།	dNgul-chu		Mercury Quicksilver	The only liquid mineral element, its nature is likened to mind and the winds. Extremely poisonous in its natural state. Said to increase vitality and longevity. G-P 13, Prec. Ess.

Tibetan Script	Tibetan Name	Latin Name	English Name	Information
ཚ་གང་	Cu-gang		Bamboo pith	Sweet substance secreted in the joints of bamboos. It cures sores and inflammations of the lungs. One of the "Six Good Things." G-Z 78, Gist 1, 12.
ཆང་	Chang		Tibetan beer	A vehicle for taking medicines. G-Z 78, 79.
སྙིང་སྣ་	sNying-sna		Various hearts	Gist 1, 13.
སྙིང་ཞོ་ཤ་	sNying-sho-sha	(a sister plant of *Canavalia gladiata*)		Good for heart ailments. The fruit or bean inside its long pod looks like a heart. Gist 1.
ཏིག་ཏ་	Tig-ta	*Gentiana barbata* *Swertia chirata* *Gentiana chiretta*	Gentian	Of three species: Indian, Tibetan and Nepalese. It cures all kinds of bilious fevers and bile diseases. Bitter. G-Z 78—twice.
རྟ་	rTa		Horse	Usually male. Here feces. G-Z 79.
སྟག་ཚེར་	sTag-tsher	*Robus idaeus* or *Solanum xanthocarpum*	Red raspberry Indian salamin	Prickly hedge berry. G-Z 78.
ཐལ་ཏྲེས་	Thal-tres	*Hemidesmus indicus*	Indian sarsaparilla	G-Z 78.

Tibetan Script	Tibetan Name	Latin Name	English Name	Information
ད་ལིས་	Da-lis	Rhododendron chrysanthum	Rhododendron	Dwarf rhododendron with fragrant leaves. Black and white varieties. Cures phlegm, gonorrhoea and gives longevity. G-Z 78.
དུག་ཉུང་	Dug-nyung	Holarrhena antidysenterica	Kurchi Conessi bark	A medicinal fruit. Stops dysentery and cures biliousness. G-Z 77.
དུར་བྱིད་	Dur-byid	Ricinus communis	Castor oil plant	A plant of purgative value, its root ejects all hot and cold diseases. G-Z 78.
དོང་ག་བ་	Dong-ga-ba	Cassia fistula or Pterosperinum acerifolium	Purging cassia	A tree; the fruit is purgative. G-Z 78.
དྲི་ཆུ	Dri-chu		Urine	Literally "fragrant water." Here, red cow's urine, or a child's urine. G-Z 78, Prec. Ess.
ལྡོང་རོས་	lDong-ros		Realgar	Yellow mineral medicine of a feminine nature. Tib. syn: "seductive-one." G-Z 77.
ན་ག་གེ་སར་	Na-ga-ge-sar Ge-sar	Mesua ferrea	Cobra's saffron	A kind of saffron from the corolla of a flower, of three kinds in Tib. medicine. G-Z 78, Gist 12.

Tibetan Script	Tibetan Name	Latin Name	English Name	Information
ཕ་རྙ	Pa-rni	Desmodium gangeticum		G-Z 78.
པི་པི་ལིང་	Pi-pi-ling	Piper longum	Long pepper	One of the "Three Hots." Cures all sickness of cold. Helps against phlegm. G-Z 77, 78—twice, 79. Gist 1, 13. Prec. Ess.
པུ་ཤེལ་རྩི་	Pu-shel-rtsi	Orchis or Vetiveria zizanoides	Orchid or Khus-khus	A parasitic orchid. Root brings up phlegm and cures vomiting. G-Z 77.
པོ་སོ་ཆ་	Po-so-cha	Sesbana grandiflora		A shrub or tree. Flowers, leaves and bark used medicinally. G-Z 78.
པྲི་ཡངྐུ	Pri-yangku	Lavandula officinalis or Callicarpa macrophylla	Lavender	A medicinal and perfume shrub. A fragrant seed, grass, cereal. Tib. syn.: "flower of the elmental spirits." G-Z 77, 78.
དཔའ་སེར་	dPa-ser			An official yellow plant of bitter taste with a root resembling a radish. Good for bile. G-Z 78.
སྤང་སྤོས་	sPang-spos	Valeriana officinalis	Valerian	Literally "meadow incense." Perennial herb, the hairy rhizomes and roots constitute the drug. Tib. syn.: "hair of the elementals." G-Z 77.

Tibetan Script	Tibetan Name	Latin Name	English Name	Information
སྤང་མ	sPang-ma			A bluish mineral. G-Z 77.
སྤོས་དཀར	sPos-dkar	Shorea robusta	Sal tree	Frankincense. The resin yields white frankincense. Psych. Incen. Gist 1, 12.
སྤྱང་ཚེར	sPyang-tsher	Carduus crispus	Plumeless thistle	Boiled extracts, especially the roots. G-Z 78.
སྤྲང	sPrang		Wild honey	An important medical essence, "essence of the flower kingdom." Reinforces the vital glow. G-Z 79.
སྤྲེ	sPre		Monkey	Here, feces. G-Z 79.
ཕོ་བ་རིལ་པོ	Pho-ba-ril-po	Piper nigrum	Black pepper	Good for digestion. G-Z 77, 78. Gist 1, 13.
བ་ཡི་འོ་མ	Ba-yi-'o-ma		Red cow's milk	G-Z 78.
བ་སེར་མཁྲིས་པ	Ba-ser-mkhris-pa		Yellow cow's bile	G-Z 79.

Tibetan Script	Tibetan Name	Latin Name	English Name	Information
བ་རུ་ར་	Ba-ru-ra	Terminalia belerica	Beleric myrobalan	One of the "Three Chief Fruits." G-Z 77, 78. Psych. Incen.
བ་ཤ་ཀ་	Ba-sha-ka	Adhatoda vasica		Shrub with yellow flowers. Good for bile and liver. G-Z 78. Gist 1.
བུ་རམ་	Bu-ram		Molasses; treacle	A vehicle for taking medicines. A medical essence, the "essence of trees." G-Z 78—twice.
བོང་ང་	Bong-nga	Aconitum	Aconite Cuckoo's cap	Seven main species grow in the Himalayas. Root of flowering plant. Poisonous. Raises heat, cures heart and mental disorders caused by excess air at heart center. Here, black aconite. Tib. syn.: *sman-chen*, "great medicine." G-Z 78—Twice. Gist 13, Prec. Ess.
བོང་ང་ནག་པོ་	Bong-nga nag-po	Aconitum napellus	Black aconite	
བོང་ང་དཀར་པོ་	Bong-nga dkar-po	Aconitum heterophyllum	White aconite	White aconite said to cure bilious fevers. G-Z 77, 78.
བོང་ང་དམར་པོ་	Bong-nga mar-po		Red aconite	G-Z 78.
བོང་ང་སེར་པོ་	Bong-nga ser-po	Curcuma zerumbet	Yellow aconite	G-Z 78.

Tibetan Script	Tibetan Name	Latin Name	English Name	Information
བྱ་ཀྲི་	Bya-kri			Possibly a bird. G-Z 77.
བྱ་རྐང་པ་	Bya-rkang-ba	Delphinium grandiflorum		A fern. Psych. Incen.
བྱ་རོག་	Bya-rog		Crow	Here, feather. G-Z 79.
བྱ་རྒོད་	Bya-rgod		Vulture	Here, feather. G-Z 79.
བྱི་ཏང་ག་	Byi-tang-ga	Erycibe paniculata		Medicinal fruit said to be effective in killing worms and improving digestion. G-Z 78.
བྱི་ལ་	Byi-la		Cat	Here, urine, feces, bile, and hair. G-Z 78. Just feces—G-Z 77.
འབྲི་	'Bri		Female yak, *dri*	Here—heart Gist 13,
དབྱི་མོང་	dByi-mong	Piper chaba		Used against delirium. G-Z 77, 78.

Tibetan Script	Tibetan Name	Latin Name	English Name	Information
སྦྲུལ་ལྤགས།	sBrul-lpags		Snake skin	Snake skin is said to cure leucoderma, the meat to prevent constipation and eye disease. Skin, G-Z 77. Skin and meat, G-Z 79.
མ་ནུ།	Ma-nu	Inula helenium	Elecampane	Roots and rhizomes. G-Z 78, Gist 1.
མར་རྙིང་།	Mar-rnying		Old butter	Old butter, preferably at least nine years old. The longer it sits, the stronger it gets in all the elements and in the essences of vitality. G-Z 77, 78, 79.
རྨ་བྱ།	rMa-bya		Peacock	Both peacock feather, the part which has the lunar rainbow design and a medicinal grass called "peacock feather." G-Z 77.
ཙན་དན་	Tsan-dan	Santalum album	Sandalwood White sandalwood	Aromatic and antiseptic. Used in medicines in many ways. Inhibits air. G-Z 77, 78—twice.
ཚི་ཏྲ་ཀ	Tsi-tra-ka	Capsicium annum or Plumbago zeylanica	Red pepper or Leadwort	A type of hot chili. G-Z 78.

Tibetan Script	Tibetan Name	Latin Name	English Name	Information
ཛཱ་ཏི	Dzaa-ti	Myristica fragrans	Nutmeg	One of the "Six Good Things." It helps correct all air imbalances and heart disease. Very important in mental disease. Tib. syn.: "King of Incenses." G-Z 78—four times. Gist 1, 12, 13. Psych. Incen. Prec. Ess.
ཝ	Wa		Tibetan Fox	Here, urine, feces, bile, nail and skin; its liver is for lung diseases. G-Z 78.
ཟེར་མོ	Zer-mo			Small yellow feathered bird with red stripes on head. Here, red and yellow feathers. G-Z 79.
འུ་སུ	'U-su	Coriandrum sativum	Coriander	Removes hot phlegm in the stomach. G-Z 78.
འུག་པ	'Ug-pa		Owl	Here, feathers, feces, and urine. G-Z 78.
ཡུང་བ	Yung-ba	Curcuma longa	Turmeric	G-Z 78—twice.
ཡུངས་དཀར	Yungs-dkar	Brassica alba	White mustard	G-Z 77.
གཡག་རྒོད	gYag-rgod		Wild yak	Heart. Gist 13, Prec. Ess.

Tibetan Script	Tibetan Name	Latin Name	English Name	Information
རྃ་ཐུག	Ra-thug		Ram	Here, urine, feces, bile, nails, hair and skin. In incenses against demonic forces. G-Z 78.
རི་བོང	Ri-bong		Rabbit	Here, heart. Prec. Ess.
རུ་རྟ	Ru-rta	Costus speciosus or Saussurea lappa		A light brown spicy root. G-Z 77, 78—twice; 79. Gist 12, Prec. Ess.
རུས་ཆེན	Rus-chen		Man's bones	Human bones should be from a young healthy person who died accidentally. G-Z 78.
རེ་རལ	Re-ral			A fern or fern root. Boiled extracts. G-Z 78.
ལ་ལ་ཕུད	La-la-phud	Trachyspermum ammi	Bishop's weed	A medicine plant. G-Z 78.
ལི་ཤི	Li-shi	Syzygium aromaticum Caryophyllus aromaticus	Clove	One of the "Six Good Things"; specifically for the life-nerve. Also for cold and liver complaints. Tib. syn.: "flower of the gods." G-Z 78—four times Gist 1, 12, 13.

Tibetan Script	Tibetan Name	Latin Name	English Name	Information
ཤ་ཆེན་	Sha-chen		"Human flesh"	From a healthy person between the ages of 16 and 30 who has died accidentally. Flesh dried for one year before use. Or, red meat or chicken meat. G-Z 78, Gist 12.
ཤིང་ཀུན་	Shing-kun	Ferula assafoetida	Asafoetida Devil's dung Food of the gods	In medicine, the strong smelling gummy juice extract from the root. One of the "Three Precious Keepers of the Life Wind." Said to cure worms, cold and heart complaints caused by excess of air. Aphrodisiac and rejuvenator. G-Z 77, Gist 1, 12.
ཤུ་དག་	Shu-dag	Acorus calamus	Sweet flag	Grows near water, on river banks, etc. Aromatic rhizome used in medicine. The black variety is indicated by the general name. G-Z 77, 78, 79. Prec. Ess.
ཤུག་པ་	Shug-pa	Juniperius pseudosabina Juniperus excelsa	Himalayan juniper	A sacred tree. Its berries are burnt as incense for delerium of fever. G-Z 77, 79. Psych. Incen.

Tibetan Script	Tibetan Name	Latin Name	English Name	Information
སུག་སྨེལ་	Sug-smel	Elettaria cardomomum	Cardamom	One of the "Six Good Things," specifically for kidney ailments. G-Z 77, 78—twice, 79. Psych. Incen., Gist 1.
སེ་འབྲུ་	Se-'bru	Punica granatum	Pomegranate	Said to cure all cold diseases and stomach problems. G-Z 77, 79.
སྲན་ཕུབ་	Sran-phub		Pease-straw	Skin of a bean. G-Z 77.
གསེར་མེ་ཏོག་	gSer-me-tog	Magnolia champaka	Yellow champa	A golden flower of Indian origin, used for bile disorders. G-Z 78.
ཧ་རི་ནུ་ཀ	Ha-ri-nu-ka	Vitex agnus-castus		A kind of pulse with fragrant but bitter medicinal substance. Good against heat. G-Z 78.
ཧོང་ལེན་	Hong-len	Picrorhiza kurroa	Hellebore	A medicinal root and rhizome, grows where snow falls. Three kinds, white, brown and yellow. Bitter and aromatic. G-Z 77, 78.

Tibetan Script	Tibetan Name	Latin Name	English Name	Information
ཨ་གུ་རུ	A-ga-ru	Aquilara agallocha	Aloeswood Eaglewood Agalloch	Especially sacred evergreen tree with occult properties. Of three varieties. Oleoresin, wood and essential oil used in medicine and incense. Scent drives away evil spirits. Here, the best—the black one; frankincense and wood. Used for mental illness. Psych. Incen. Gist 1, 12, 13. Pres. Ess.
ཨ་གུ་རུ་ནག་པོ	A-ga-ru-nag-po			
ཨར་སྐྱ	Ar-skya	Boswellia serrata	Indian frankincense tree	The grey-white aloeswood and frankincense. Psych. Incen.
ཨར་དམར	Ar-dmar		Red aloeswood	The red aloeswood and frankincense. Psych. Incen.
ཨ་རུ་ར	A-ru-ra	Terminalia chebula	Chebulic myrobalan Myrobalan	Seven varieties. Each part of this tree used for different ailments. Emblem of the Medicine Buddha. Tib. syn: "Supreme Medicine," "Universal Medicine." G-Z 78—twice. Prec. Ess.
ཨུཏྤ་ལ ཏྣ་ཌུ་ཏ་པ་ལ	Ut-pala or Dan-da-u-ta-pa-la	Nymphaea stellata	Blue lotus	Root and flowering lotus plant. Increases fertility. G-Z 78. Gist 1.

Appendix II

Summary of the
Four Tantras of rGyud-bzhi*

I. *rTsa-rgyud* (Root Tantra) Six Chapters
   1. Basic discussion of history: How the Buddha transformed into the Medicine Buddha and gave this teaching
   2. Cause of discussion
   3. Basics of disease—Simile of the "Tree of Health and Disease"
   4. Examinations of disease—symptoms
   5. Treatment
   6. Recapitulation of the above

II. *bShad-rgyud* (Commentary Tantra) Thirty-one Chapters
   1. Summarized explanation of medicine
   2. Embryology
   3. Anatomy (in similes)
   4. Physiology
   5. Characterization of the body
   6. Types of body and their functioning
   7. Signs of approaching death
   8. The seeds (causes) of disease
   9. Accessory causes of disease
   10. Ways of entrance of disease

*Based on combined sources, mainly the teachings of Dr. Pema Dorje and the outline of Csoma de Koros.

11. Symptoms, character of disease
12. Classification of diseases
13. Everyday conduct
14. Conduct during the seasons
15. Occasional and general conduct, avoidance of obstructing natural impulses
16. Food and drink
17. Dietary rules, harmful combinations of food
18. Right quantities of food and drink
19. Taste and digestive qualities of medicines, preparing medicine
20. Materia medica
21. Pharmacology, specification
22. Surgical instruments
23. Health rules
24. Diagnosis of humoral diseases
25. Vicious mental inclinations as causes of diseases
26. Doctor, nurse and patient
27. General rules of healing
28. How to begin the treatment of particular diseases
29. How to improve and maintain good health, fasts and diets
30. Humoral pathology and treatment
31. Required qualities and duties of a doctor

III. *Man-ngag rgyud* (Pith Instruction Tantra)
Ninety-two chapters
1. Introduction—manner of curing diseases
2. Diseases of air
3. Diseases of bile
4. Diseases of phlegm
5. Integration of air, bile, and phlegm
6. Indigestion
7. Abdominal tumor
8. First stage of dropsy
9. Second stage of dropsy
10. Full dropsy
11. Tuberculosis
12. General fevers
13. Causes of heat in fever
14. Causes of cold in fever
15. Unripened fever

16. Fully mature fever
17. Empty or latent fever
18. Hidden fever
19. Chronic fever
20. Mixed fever
21. Spreading fever
22. Disturbed fever
23. Infectious fever, diseases, and epidemics
24. Small pox
25. Colic
26. Scarlet fever, throat swellings and ulcers
27. Catarrh
28. Head diseases
29. Eye diseases
30. Ear diseases
31. Nose diseases
32. Mouth diseases
33. Goiter and throat diseases
34. Heart diseases
35. Lung diseases
36. Liver diseases
37. Spleen diseases
38. Kidney diseases
39. Stomach diseases
40. Small intestine diseases
41. Large intestine diseases
42. Male genital diseases
43. Female genital diseases
44. Hoarseness
45. Anorexia
46. Thirst
47. Hiccough
48. Asthma
49. Acute abdominal pains
50. Worm diseases
51. Vomiting
52. Diarrhea
53. Constipation
54. Urinary retention
55. Frequent urination
56. Dysentery (called "Indian Heat sickness")

57. Gout
58. Rheumatism
59. Jaundice
60. Paralysis, "the white vein"
61. Skin disorders
62. Minor diseases
63. Congenital adenopathy
64. Piles
65. Ringworm
66. Cancerous sores
67. Tumors
68. Swelling of the testicles
69. Elephantiasis
70. Rectal abcess
71. Midwifery, infant diseases
72. Childhood diseases
73. Fifteen evil spirits causing nervous diseases in children
74. Gynaecology
75. Special gynaecology
76. Common female problems
77. Insanity through possession by elemental spirits
78. Spirits causing madness
79. Spirits causing loss of memory
80. Planetary demons causing epilepsy and paralysis
81. Serpent-spirits causing leprosy and emaciation of the body in chronic mental diseases
82. General wounds, injuries
83. Head wounds
84. Neck injuries
85. Abdominal wounds
86. Limb wounds
87. Purposely compounded poisons
88. Food poisoning
89. Plant, animal and mineral poisons
90. Rejuvenation treatment for the aged, senile feebleness
91. Treatment for impotence, support for the senile person
92. Treatment for infertility, strengthening the aging organism

IV. *Phyi-ma-rgyud* (Last Tantra) Twenty-seven chapters
   1. Pulse examination
   2. Urine examination

3. Decoction (herbal teas)—77 kinds
4. Powdered medicines—165 kinds
5. Pills—22 kinds
6. Condensed paste medicines with sweetener—20 kinds
7. Medicinal butter—23 kinds
8. Ashes of metals as medicines—13 kinds
9. Condensed decoctions, syrups—17 kinds
10. Medicinal liquids or wines—19 kinds
11. Precious medicines from jewels and metals—20 kinds
12. Herbal medicines—28 for heat, 14 for cold, 416 altogether mentioned
13. Treatment by oil taken orally for purging
14. Purgation—82 kinds of medicine
15. Therapeutic vomiting, emetics
16. Nose cleaning medicines—16 kinds
17. Enemas of extracted juices
18. Use of instrument to insert medicine in colon
19. "Washing nerves," elixirs for cleansing the channels
20. Bloodletting for hot diseases—77 veins
21. Moxibustion—for cold diseases
22. Applying hot and cold compresses at pain sights, use of venomous mixtures
23. Medicinal baths
24. Massage and medicinal ointments
25. "Spoon"—method of extracting accumulation of fluid between heart and pericardium, medicines operating downwards, surgical treatments
26. Conclusion: Condensing the 1,200 ways of examining diseases into three ways
27. Classification and moral application of the above 404 diseases

Notes

Part I

1. Additionally, the Centre has a pharmacy, research department, and museum. Underfunded, it supports its charitable hospital and other works by the sale of traditional Tibetan medicines and other products. Information may be obtained by writing the Director, Tibetan Medical Centre, Dharamsala, H.P. India.

2. Shantideva, *A Guide to the Bodhisattva's Way of Life,* trans. Stephen Batchelor (Dharamsala, India: Library of Tibetan Works and Archives, 1979), p. 179. Used by permission.

3. Jhampa Kelsang, trans., *The Ambrosia Heart Tantra* (the *rGyud-bzhi*) Vol. I (Dharamsala, India: Library of Tibetan Works and Archives, 1977), p. 76. Used by permission.

4. See Franz Alexander and Sheldon Selesnick, *The History of Psychiatry* (New York: Harper & Row, 1966), pp. 26-34.

5. Theodore Burang, *The Tibetan Art of Healing,* trans. Susan Macintosh (London: Robinson & Watkins Books, Ltd., 1974), p. 89. Used by permission.

6. Elizabeth Finckh, *Foundations of Tibetan Medicine,* trans. Fredericka M. Houser, Vol. I (London: Robinson & Watkins Books, Ltd., 1978).

7. Along with Vaidya Bhagwan Dash's translation of Nagarjuna's *Yogasataka* (*sByor-ba brgya-pa*) or the *Hundred Prescriptions* is a history of Indo-Tibetan medicine and an index of Tibetan medical terms; Dharamsala, 1976. Also see Claus Vogel's

translation of the first five chapters of the Tibetan version of Vagbhata's *Astangahridayasamhita* (Wiesbaden, 1965), which also still exists in the original Sanskrit.

8. New books and a journal on Tibetan medicine are expected from the Library of Tibetan Works and Archives (LTWA) in Dharamsala, H.P., India. One is also due from the Tibetan Medical Centre.

9. Edward Conze, ed. and trans., *Buddhist Scriptures* (London: Penguin Classics, 1959), pp. 187, 189. Copyright © 1959 by Edward Conze. Reprinted by permission of Penguin Books, Ltd.

10. *Ibid.,* p. 187.

11. Edward Conze, *Buddhist Meditation* (London: George Allen & Unwin, Ltd., 1956), pp. 17-18. Used by permission.

12. Based primarily on the teaching of His Holiness Dudjom Rinpoche, head of the Nyingmapa school of Tibetan Buddhism.

13. From the commentary to "Songs of the Sisters," cited by Ananda Nimalasuria, ed., *Buddha the Healer* (Kandy: Buddhist Publication Society, 1960), p. 7.

14. Early translation (from a French translation) by Henry D. Thoreau in *The Dial,* Vol. IV (3), 1884.

15. *Entering the Path of Enlightenment,* trans. by Marion L. Matics, Macmillan Publishing Co., Inc., New York, and Allen & Unwin, Ltd., London. Used by permission.

16. Cited by Heinrich Zimmer, *Philosophies of India,* ed. Joseph Campbell (New York: Meridian, 1951), p. 522.

17. *Ibid.,* p. 523.

18. *Crystal Mirror,* Vol. IV (Berkeley, CA: Dharma Publishing, 1975), pp. 124-125. Used by permission.

19. Geshe Rabten, cited by Janice D. Willis, *The Diamond Light of the Eastern Dawn* (New York: Simon & Schuster, 1971), p. 37. Used by permission.

20. Cited by Blanche Olschak, "Traditional Therapies of Ancient India" (*Sandoz News,* 3, 1966), p. 15.

21. Charles Leslie, ed., *Asian Medical Systems* (Berkeley, CA: University of California Press, 1976), p. 7.

22. Heinrich Zimmer, *Hindu Medicine* (Baltimore: The Johns Hopkins Press, 1948), p. 52.

23. *Ibid.,* p. 50.

24. Because of the conceptual differences held by Western and Eastern authorities about the dates of past historical times and because of the recurrence of names of historical figures in

different centuries, there is a widely divergent dating of Charaka *et al.* For example, Sylvan Levi places Charaka about the 2nd century A.D., while Bhagwan Dash places him at 600 B.C. For fuller discussion of this controversy see O.P. Jaggi, *Indian System of Medicine* (Delhi: Atma Ram & Sons, 1973), pp. 12-15.

25. Cited by Nimalasuria, *op. cit.,* p. 32.

26. A. L. Basham, "The Practice of Medicine in Ancient and Medieval India," *Asian Medical Systems,* ed. Charles Leslie (Berkeley, CA: University of California Press, 1976), p. 24.

27. Zimmer, *Hindu Medicine,* p. 32.

28. Jyotir Mitra, "Lord Buddha—A Great Physician," *Religion and Medicine,* ed. K. N. Udupa (Varanasi, India: Institute of Medical Sciences, BHU, 1974), pp. 50-51.

29. Cited by Alschak, *op. cit.,* p. 14.

30. Pierre Huard and Ming Wong, *Chinese Medicine* (New York: McGraw-Hill Book Co., 1968), p. 91.

31. According to the Tibetans, Ashvaghosha and Vagbhata are the same person; that is, he is known to the Indians as Vagbhata and to the Tibetans as Ashvaghosha. Most of the great Indian saints had many names by which they were known.

32. Mitra, *op. cit.,* p. 53.

33. Cited by Dasgupta, *Obscure Religious Cults,* 3rd ed. (Calcutta: Mukhopadhyay, 1969), p. 89.

34. Boiled water is still a basic remedy of Tibetan medicine for all manner of digestive complaints. It must be boiled for at least twenty minutes; some prescriptions call for longer and repeated boilings to bring water to a state of purified liquid essence.

35. The eight Medicine Buddhas are: *mTshan-legs-yongs-grags-dpal; sGra-dbyangs-rgyal-po; gSer-bzang-dri-med-rin-chen-snang; Myang-ngan-med- mchog-dpal; Chos-grags-rgya-mtsho'i-dbyangs; mNgon-mkhyen-rgyal-po; rGyal-ba-seng-ge'i-nga-ro; Rin-chen-gtsug-tor-chen.*

36. There are eight medicine goddesses: *bDud-rtsi-ma; Grub-pa'i-lha-mo; gZe-brjid-lha-mo; 'Od-ljag; rMug-bsel; gDong-Khra-ma; mDangs-ldan; Rigs-byed-ma.*

37. Rechung Rinpoche, *Tibetan Medicine* (Berkeley, CA: University of California Press, 1973), p. 180. Copyright © 1973 by The Wellcome Trust. Reprinted by permission of University of California Press, Berkeley, CA, and The Wellcome Institute for the History of Medicine, London.

38. The Persian doctor's name "Galenos" was no doubt adopted as a tribute to the great Greek physician Galen, since Persian medicine incorporated and preserved the ancient system of classical Greek medicine. This serves to emphasize that the medical learning of the Greeks found its way into the Tibetan tradition.

39. Specifically, he took it from the Vase Pillar of the Central Hall of the Upper Shrine at Samye at approximately 1:12 A.M. on the 15th day, 7th month, earth male tiger year, then copied the book and returned it to its proper resting place; according to H.H. Dudjom Rinpoche, *Nyingmapa History*, translated by Gyurmed Dorje and Matthew Kapstein (unpublished manuscript).

40. V. Bhagwan Dash, "Indian Contribution to Tibetan Medicine," *An Introduction to Tibetan Medicine*, ed. Dawa Norbu (Delhi: Tibetan Review Publications, 1976), p. 13.

41. Charles Leslie, "The Ambiguities of Medical Revivalism in Modern India," *op. cit.*, pp. 356-367.

42. Because of Mongolian Ayurveda the Russians have shown a keen interest in Tibetan medicine. Czar Alexander I commissioned a translation of the *rGyud-bzhi* (never completed), and top modern Russian scientists and scholars at the Academy of Sciences of the USSR have produced the most thorough scientific studies yet on Tibetan medicine.

43. Pierre Huard and Ming Wong, *op. cit.*, p. 112.

44. Rechung, *op. cit.*, p. 26.

45. David Snellgrove and Hugh Richardson, *A Cultural History of Tibet* (New York: Frederick A. Praeger, 1968), p. 262.

46. Garma C. C. Chang, *The Teachings of Tibetan Yoga* (New Hyde Park, NY: University Books, 1963), p. 116.

47. Drashi Namjhal, "Introduction to the Profound Path of the Six Yogas," *Teachings of Tibetan Yoga*, p. 118.

48. Tulu Thondup, *A Summary of Mipham Rinpoche's Commentary on The Seven Line Prayer* (Providence, RI: Mahasiddha Nyingmapa Center, 1977). Used by permission.

49. William Stablein, "Tibetan Medical-Cultural System," *An Introduction to Tibetan Medicine*, ed. Dawa Norbu (Delhi: Tibetan Review Publications, 1976), pp. 39-51.

50. Mircea Eliade, *Patanjali and Yoga* (New York: Schocken Books, 1976), p. 183.

51. The foregoing description is based on the teachings of Dodrup Chen Rinpoche.

52. Tulku Thonup, trans., *Instructions on Turning Suffering and Happiness into the Path of Enlightenment* (Darjeeling, India: Ogyan Kunsang Choekhorling Monastery, 1979), p. 5. Used by permission.

53. This meditation and mantra may be practiced without initiation. However, if one can receive the transmission and initiation from a qualified lineage-holder, it is recommended to do so.

54. That is the Tibetan pronunciation. The actual Sanskrit pronunciation is: TADYATHA OM BHAISHAJYA BHAISHAJ-YA MAHABHAISHAJYA BHAISHAJARATA SAMUDGATE SVAHA.

55. Pema Dorje, a young English-speaking Tibetan doctor who teaches at the Tibetan Medical School at Dharamsala, India.

56. According to different lamas and teachings, the seats of the life-bearing wind and the pervasive wind can be reversed: the life-bearing wind can be said to be seated in the head and the pervasive wind to be at the heart. The reason they have a reciprocal character and can be switched is because the white thigle in the head center comes from the central primary thigle in the heart, and both these thigles support consciousness throughout the body; thus, both the head and the heart relate to mental functioning.

57. Mainly based on Csoma de Koros's outline of the *Gyu-zhi*, "Analysis of a Tibetan Medical Work," *Journal of the Asiatic Society of Bengal*, 4, 1835, pp. 1-20.

58. Rechung, *op. cit.*, pp. 96-97.

59. *Ibid.*

60. Yeshi Dhonden and Jeffrey Hopkins, "An Anatomy of Body and Disease," *An Introduction to Tibetan Medicine*, ed. Dawa Norbu (Delhi: Tibetan Review Publications, 1976), pp. 28-29. Reprinted courtesy of Jeffrey Hopkins.

61. This is called attaining the "rainbow body" (*'ja-lus*), in which the inner elements of the body are transmuted into their most subtle counterparts, which appear as five-colored lights. Only the nails and hair remain. This is an actual tradition in Tibet, and there are said to be uncountable numbers of saints who have attained this level—even in recent history.

62. W. Y. Evans-Wentz, trans., *The Tibetan Book of the Dead* (New York: Oxford University Press, 1960), pp. xxxvi-xxxvii.

63. Rechung, *op. cit.*, p. 32.

64. *The Jewel Ornament of Liberation* by sGam Po Pa, trans. by Herbert V. Guenther, published by Rider Books, a part of the

Hutchinson Publishing Group (1959), p. 65. Used by permission.

65. Rechung, *op. cit.,* p. 37.
66. *Ibid.,* p. 57.
67. *Ibid.*

Part II

1. The eight branches of Tibetan medicine, which are slightly different from the eight of classical Indian Ayurveda, are: physical ailments, women's ailments, wounds inflicted by weapons, children's ailments, ailments caused by spirits, ailments caused by poisons, ailments of the aged, and sterility.

2. Dr. Ama Lobsang, Chief Physician, Tibetan Medical Centre, Dharamsala, India.

3. *Op. cit.,* p. 19.

4. As described in the Second Tantra, Rechung, *op. cit.,* p. 40.

5. Dhonden and Hopkins, *op. cit.,* p. 25.

6. Compare this to the shamanic model in which the prime candidate for training as a shaman or wiseman is the youngster who exhibits a psychotic personality. See Eliade's monumental work *Shamanism.*

7. According to Dr. Ama Lobsang.

8. The Tibetan system starts the counting of vertebrae from the highest prominent vertebra at the base of the neck, which corresponds to the seventh cervical in the Western system.

9. *The Diagnostic and Statistical Manual of Mental Disorders (DSM II)* (Washington, DC: American Psychiatric Association, 1968), pp. 33-34.

10. *Ibid.*

11. Patrul Rinpoche, "Instructions on How to Become Victorious over Demons by Abandoning Them and Checking Their Origins," *The Collected Works of dPal-sprul O'rgyan 'Jigs-med Chos-Kyi dBang-po,* Vol. II (Gangtok, Sikkim: Sonam Topgay Kazi, 1970), folios 639-673.

12. Ma-Chig-la, "Demons: Routing the Forces of Obstruction," *Gesar,* III (1) (Berkeley, CA: Dharma Publishing, 1975), p. 6. Used by permission.

13. Burang, *op. cit.,* p. 92.

14. The etymology according to Professor R.A.F. Thurman, Amherst College.

15. Cited by Morton Kelsey, *Discernment: A Study in Ecstasy* (New York: Paulist Press, 1978), p. 77.

16. *The Hundred Thousand Songs of Milarepa,* translated and annotated by Garma C.C. Chang (University Books, 1962), p. 5. Published by arrangement with University Books, Inc., a division of Lyle Stuart, Inc. Used by permission.

17. Reprinted by special arrangement with Shambhala Publications, Inc., 1920 13th Street, Boulder, Colorado 80302. From *Cutting Through Spiritual Materialism* © 1973 by Chögyam Trungpa; p. 241.

18. Burang, *op. cit.,* p. 90.

19. This information on formation of ghosts is based on teachings of Tulku Pema Wangyal. Interestingly, American psychic research on the history of ghosts and cases of haunting shows that almost all ghosts occur in connection with suicides, murders, and "unfinished business."

20. Just to emphasize how much classification varies with various Tibetan traditions, a book called the *White Umbrella* says there are 420 *gdon* rather than the 360 *gdon* mentioned by R. Nebesky-Wojkowitz in *Oracles and Demons of Tibet.* (London: Oxford Press, 1959), the most comprehensive work on this subject. The *White Umbrella* also gives names of the various deities who protect against each specific *gdon* and much similar information. It has not yet been translated from Tibetan.

21. A star leaving a tail of green smoke behind it is a *gZaa-yi-gdon,* according to Dodrup Chen Rinpoche.

22. According to Burang, the days of the lunar month on which epileptic seizures occur are: 4th, 8th, 11th, 15th (full moon), 18th, 22nd, 25th, and 29th.

    As for outer "radiating effects" causing leprosy, it is interesting to note that certain types of epileptic seizures are set off by those ubiquitous "demons"—television and fluorescent lights and the frequency of their flickers.

23. Here Garuda symbolized absolute wisdom, the naga-snake ignorance, and leprosy the results of ignorance. Of course, leprosy is a contagious disease caused by a strain of bacteria that lives in the ground (which may be, in fact, what the "demons from below" represent).

24. This channel in the ring finger is associated with the rise of negative emotions. As a protective measure against contracting "demons" and the destructive emotions that inflame the mind, one is supposed to press down with the thumb on the inside base of the ring finger.

Lamas have also said that, once possessed, if one ties the base of the ring finger with a blessed string, the demon will feel trapped and will begin to reveal through the patient's words and actions who and what he is and where he came from.

25.   Patrul Rinpoche, *op. cit.,* folios 207-210.

26.   This is the opinion of Yeshe Dorje Rinpoche, rainmaker and exorcist.

27.   Longchenpa, *Kindly Bent to Ease Us,* trans. H.V. Guenther, Vol. II (Berkeley, CA: Dharma Publishing, 1976), p. 48.

28.   Cited by Gampopa, *op. cit.,* p. 223.

29.   Reprinted by special arrangement with Shambhala Publications, Inc.., 1920 13th Street, Boulder, Colorado 80302. From *Treasures on the Tibetan Middle Way* by Herbert V. Guenther (1969), p. 223.

30.   *Ibid.,* pp. 36-37.

31.   This foregoing classification of different types of exorcism is based on the teaching of Doboom Rinpoche, Director, Library of Tibetan Works and Archives, Dharamsala, India.

32.   W. Y. Evans-Wentz, trans., "The Path of the Mystic Sacrifice," *Tibetan Yoga and Secret Doctrines,* 2nd ed. (New York: Oxford University Press, 1967), p. 317. Used by permission.

33.   Pareshnath, trans., *Charaka-Samhita,* Vol. III (Calcutta: P. Sarma, 1906).

34.   The translation was done by Ven. Namdrol Gyamtso and Lodro Thaye and is based primarily on the oral instructions and explication of the Tibetan lama-doctor Dodrag Amchi of KSL Monastery, Bodhnath, Nepal. The Scottish yogi Gyurmed-Dorje helped make the preliminary translation. Ven. Geshe Jamspal of the Buddhist Institute of New Jersey made a final reading with corrections.

35.   Why possession by the five "great elementals" precedes the full blown psychosis described in relation to the eighteen elementals as a general group is unclear. One possible interpretation is that those five, all of which are related to higher spiritual life, represent the attempt to advance spiritually and to break out of the confines of ordinary mentality. In this sense they may represent some kind of insight and heightened consciousness that goes awry, spiritual development that goes in the wrong direction, and consequently mind, having been opened up to vaster dimensions, is unable to integrate the experiences in a positive way and is subsequently overcome by them. This relates

to the idea that insanity and spiritual advancement are the two possibilities that follow from insight into reality.

Another possible interpretation regards the following correspondence: In Buddhist philosophy there are "five great elements," which are sometimes described as sub-atomic cosmic-physical principles, and there are the "eighteen elements" which express the functioning of ordinary consciousness—six dominant elements or sense organs, including mind; six sense elements, or the activity of the senses, including thought; and six object elements. When the five great elements (*'byung-ba,* the same word root as elemental spirits— *'byung-po'i gdon,* literally spirits of the elements) are disturbed by mind and emotion, then this can be interpreted as a disturbance of the basic biochemical ground that subsequently gives rise to eighteen basic divisions of perceptual distortions and disturbed consciousness.

36. *DSM II, op. cit.,* p. 34.
37. *Ibid.,* p. 33.
38. Anila Yangchen-la and Chos-kyi-la of the OKC Monastery in Darjeeling translated for Lama Wangla, explained the text, procured the ingredients for the medicine, and assisted in the making of it.
39. Perhaps nowhere is this transformational aspect of medicine more clear than in the processing of mercury. Mercury is said to be like the mind. It is mobile and fluid, highly volatile. It is also a deadly poison in its ordinary state. When stabilized and purified, it becomes the most powerful elixir—like mind in its realized state.

 The actual Tibetan process of purifying mercury for medicines is extremely difficult and takes at least three days to complete, using numerous ingredients in a specific ratio and manner. It involves, in part, mixing the raw mercury with a fern root and wild ginger, placing these together in a piece of soft musk leather, which is tightly tied with a cord so that the ingredients are in a little sack. The bag is rubbed in the palm of the hand for one day, long enough for the herbal mixture to draw out and absorb the mercury's poisons. The leather also absorbs them. When taken out, the herb mixture has turned black and the mercury looks much cleaner and shinier than before.

 After a few more intermediate stages, the mercury is

boiled in cow's urine with more purifying herbs, salts, and metals. At subsequent stages the mercury is cooked in oil and combined with powdered sulphur that has itself been through a purifying process. In combination with mercury, the poisonous effects of both are further counteracted. Finally, a yellow powder results. It is ground without stopping for a day and a half until it turns into an extremely fine pitch-black powder.

40. Translated from *The Gist Prescriptions of the Traditional Tibetan Medicines* (Dharamsala, India: Tibetan Medical Centre, 1972), pp. 7-12.

41. Burang, *op. cit.,* pp. 47-48.

42. Cited by Alexander and Selesnick, *op. cit.,* p. 352.

43. Erich Fromm, *Psychoanalysis and Religion* (New York: Bantam Books, 1950), p. 76.

44. Francis Story, "Buddhist Mental Therapy," in Nimalasuria, *op. cit.,* p. 30.

45. Work applying the principles of Buddhist psychology to modern clinical psychology has been done in America by Tarthang Tulku Rinpoche at the Nyingma Institute in Berkeley, California, and Chogyam Trungpa Rinpoche at the Naropa Institute in Boulder, Colorado.

46. Herbert Fingarette, *The Self in Transformation* (New York: Basic Books, 1963), p. 180.

47. Alexander and Selesnick, *op. cit.,* pp. 47-48.

48. Renchung, *op. cit.,* p. 32.

49. W. Y. Evans-Wentz translation in *The Tibetan Book of the Great Liberation* (New York: Oxford University Press, 1954) pp. 215, 220, 228. Used by permission.

Bibliography

Books and Articles

Ackerknecht, Erwin. *A Short History of Medicine*. Rev. ed. New York: The Roland Press Co., 1968.

Alexander, F. and S. Selesnick. *The History of Psychiatry*. New York: Harper & Row, 1966.

The Ambrosia Heart Tantra: The Secret Oral Teaching on the Eight Branches of the Science of Healing, Vol. I. Annotated by Yeshi Donden. Translated by Jhampa Kelsang. Dharamsala: Library of Tibetan Works and Archives, 1977.

Bai Dur sNgon Po (The Lapis Lazuli Commentary on the rGyud-bzhi) of Sangs-rgyas rGya-mtsho. Leh, Ladakh: T. Y. Tashigangpa, 1973, Vol. 3.

Bajra, Mana. *An Outline of Ayurveda*. Kathmandu: Piyusavarsi Ausah-hala, 1975.

Beau, Georges. *Chinese Medicine*. Trans. Lowell Bair. New York: Avon Books, 1972.

Bharati, Agehananda. *The Tantric Tradition*. Rev. ed., New York: Samuel Weiser, Inc., 1975.

Bhattacharyya Benoytosh. *Gem Therapy*. 2nd ed., Calcutta: Mukho-padhyay, 1971.

Birnbaum, Raoul. *The Healing Buddha*. Boulder: Shambhala, 1979.

Blofeld, John. *The Tantric Mysticism of Tibet*. New York: E. P. Dutton & Co., 1970.

————. *The Wheel of Life.* Rpt., Berkeley: Shambhala, 1972.

Burang, Theodore. *The Tibetan Art of Healing.* Trans. Susan Macintosh. London: Robinson & Watkins Books Ltd., 1974.

Burtt, Edwin A. *The Teachings of the Compassionate Buddha.* New York: Mentor Books, 1955.

Chandra, Lokesh, ed. *An Illustrated Tibeto-Mongolian Materia Medica of Ayurveda of 'Jam-dpal-rdo-rje of Mongolia.* New Delhi: International Academy of Indian Culture, 1971.

Chang, Garma C. C. *The Hundred Thousand Songs of Milarepa.* Abridged edition. New York: Harper Colophon Books, 1970.

————. *The Teachings of Tibetan Yoga.* New Hyde Park, N.Y.: University Books, 1963.

Charaka-Samhita. Trans. Pareshnath Sarma. Calcutta: P. Sarma, 1906. Vol. 3.

Chen, C. M. *Discriminations Between Buddhist and Hindu Tantras.* Kalimpong, India: C. M. Chen, 1969.

————. *The Practice of Sunyata in the Hinayana, Mahayana, and Vajrayana.* Trans. Jivata. Kalimpong, India: C. M. Chen, 1972.

Chinese Medicinal Herbs. Comp. Li Shih-Chen. Trans. F. Porter Smith and G.A. Stuart. San Francisco: Georgetown Press, 1973.

Chopra, Ram Nath. *Indigenous Drugs of India.* Calcutta: Art Press, 1933.

Conze, Edward. *Buddhist Meditation.* London: George Allen & Unwin, Ltd., 1956.

————, trans. and ed. *Buddhist Scriptures.* London: Penguin Books, 1959.

————. *Buddhist Wisdom Books.* London: Allen & Unwin, 1958.

Csoma, de Koros, Alexander. "Analysis of a Tibetan Medical Work." *Journal of the Asiatic Society of Bengal.* (Jan., 1835), pp. 1-20.

Dargyay, Eva M. *The Rise of Esoteric Buddhism in Tibet.* Delhi: Motilal Banarsidass, 1977.

Das, Sarat Chandra. *A Tibetan English Dictionary.* 1902; rpt. Delhi: Motilal Banarsidass, 1970.

Dasgupta, S. *Obscure Religious Cults.* 3rd ed. Calcutta: Mukhopadhyay, 1969.

Dash, Vaidya Bhagwan. "The Drug *Terminalia Chebula* in Ayurveda and Tibetan Medical Literature." *Kailash, A Journal of Himalayan Studies,* 4, (1976), 5-20.

————. "Indian Contribution to Tibetan Medicine." *An Introduction to Tibetan Medicine.* Ed. Dawa Norbu. Delhi: Tibetan Review Publications, 1976.

———. "Saffron in Ayurveda and Tibetan Medicine." *The Tibet Journal,* I, (April-June, 1976), 59-66.

———. *Tibetan Medicine: With Special Reference to Yoga Sataka.* Dharamsala: Library of Tibetan Works and Archives, 1976.

Dastur, J. F. *Medicinal Plants of India and Pakistan.* Bombay: D. B. Taraporevala Sons & Co., Ltd., 1962.

Dhonden, Yeshi and Jeffrey Hopkins. "An Anatomy of Body and Disease." *An Introduction to Tibetan Medicine.* Ed. Dawa Norbu. Delhi: Tibetan Review Publications, 1976.

———, and Gyatsho Tshering. "What is Tibetan Medicine?" *An Introduction to Tibetan Medicine.* Ed. D. Norbu. Delhi: Tibetan Review Publications, 1976.

The Diagnostic and Statistical Manual of Mental Disorders (D.S.M.II). 3rd ed. Washington, D.C.: American Psychiatric Association, 1968.

Dodrup Chen Rinpoche, the 3rd. *Instructions for Turning Suffering and Happiness into the Path of Enlightenment.* Trans. Tulku Thondup. Darjeeling: Ogyan Kiunsang Choekhorling Monastery, 1979.

Eliade, Mircea. *Patanjali and Yoga.* New York: Schocken Books, 1976.

———. *Yoga: Immortality and Freedom.* Bollingen Series, LVI. Princeton Univ. Press, 1958.

Evans-Wentz, W. Y. *The Tibetan Book of the Dead.* Trans. with Lama Kazi Dawa Samdup. 3rd ed., 1957; rpt. New York: Oxford Univ. Press, 1960.

———. *The Tibetan Book of the Great Liberation.* New York: Oxford Univ. Press, 1954.

———. *Tibetan Yoga and Secret Doctrines.* Trans. with Lama Kazi Dawa Samdup. 2nd ed., 1958; rpt. New York: Oxford Univ. Press, 1967.

Filliozat, J. *The Classical Doctrine of Indian Medicine.* Delhi: Munshiram Manoharlal, 1965.

Finckh, Elisabeth. *Foundations of Tibetan Medicine,* Vol. I. Trans. Fredericka M. Houser. London: Robinson & Watkins, 1978.

Fingarette, Herbert. *The Self in Transformation.* New York: Basic Books, 1963.

Fromm, Erich. *Psychoanalysis and Religion.* New York: Bantam Books (1950), 1972.

Gammerman, A.F. and B.V. Semichov. *Slovar' tibetsko-latino-russkikh nazvanii lekarstvennogo rastitel'nogo syr'ia primenyaemogo v tibetskoi meditsine.* (Index of Tibetan Pharmacology.) Ulan Ude: Akademiya Nauk SSSR, 1963.

sGam Go Pa. *The Jewel Ornament of Liberation.* Trans. H. V. Guenther, 1959, rpt. Berkeley: Shambhala, 1971.

Gist Prescriptions of the Tibetan Traditional Medicines. Dharamsala, India: Tibetan Medical Centre, 1972.

Grousset, Rene. *In the Footsteps of the Buddha.* Trans. J.A. Underwood. New York: Grossman Publishers, 1971.

———. *Philosophy and Psychology in the Abhidharma.* 3rd ed. Berkeley: Shambhala, 1976.

Guenther, H. V. *The Royal Song of Saraha: A Study in the History of Buddhist Thought.* Berkeley: Shambhala, 1973.

———. *Treasures on the Tibetan Middle Way.* Berkeley: Shambhala, 1969.

rGyud'bźi: A Reproduction of a set of prints from the 18th century Zung-cu-ze blocks from the collection of Prof. Raghu Vira. by O-rgyan Namgyal. Leh, Ledakh: S. W. Tashigangpa, 1975.

Huard, Pierre and Ming Wong. *Chinese Medicine.* New York: McGraw-Hill Book Co., 1968.

Hunt, R. *The Seven Keys to Color Healing.* Ashington, England: C. W. Daniel and Co., 1968.

Jaggi, O. P. *Indian System of Medicine.* Delhi: Atma Ram & Sons, 1973.

———. *Yogic and Tantric Medicine.* Delhi: Atma Ram & Sons, 1973.

Jain, S. K. *Medicinal Plants.* Delhi: National Book Trust of India, 1968.

Kadans, Joseph. *Encyclopedia of Medicinal Herbs.* New York: Arco Books, 1973.

Kelsey, Morton. *Discernment: A Study in Ecstasy.* New York: Paulist Press, 1978.

Lati Rinbochay and Jeffrey Hopkins. *Death, Intermediate State and Rebirth in Tibetan Buddhism.* London: Rider and Company, 1979.

Leslie, Charles, ed. *Asian Medical Systems.* Berkeley: Univ. of California Press, 1976.

———. "The Ambiguities of Medical Revivalism of Modern India." *Asian Medical Systems.* Ed. C. Leslie. Berkley: Univ. of California Press, 1976.

Longchenpa. *Kindly Bent to Ease Us.* Trans. H. V. Guenther. Emeryville, Ca.: Dharma Publishing, 1975, 1976. 3 Vols.

———. "The Natural Freedom of Mind." *Crystal Mirror,* IV (1975), pp. 113-146.

Ma-Chig-la. "Demons: Routing the Forces of Obstruction." *Gesar,* III, (1976), 6-9.

Matics, Marion, trans. *Entering the Path of Enlightenment: The Bodhicaryavatara of the Buddhist Poet Santideva.* New York: Macmillan, 1970.

Maury, Marguerite. *The Secret of Life and Youth.* Trans. Mervyn Savill. London: MacDonald, 1964.

Medicinal Plants of Nepal. Kathmandu: H. M. G. Press, 1970.

Mipham Rinpoche. *Collected Writings of 'Jam-mgon 'Ju Mi-pham rGya-mtsho.* Gangtok, Sikkim: Sonam Topgay Kazi, 1975. Vol. 9.

Mitra, Jyotir. "Lord Buddha—A Great Physician." *Religion and Medicine.* Ed. K. N. Udupa. Varanasi, India: Institute of Medical Sciences, BHU, 1974.

Nebesky-Wojkowitz, R. *Oracles and Demons of Tibet.* London: Oxford Press, 1959.

Nimalasuria, Ananda, ed. *Buddha The Healer: The Mind and its Place in Buddhism.* Kandy, Ceylon: Buddhist Publication Society, 1960.

Norbu, Dawa, ed. *An Introduction to Tibetan Medicine.* Delhi: Tibetan Review Publications, 1976.

Olschak, Blanche. "The Art of Healing in Ancient Tibet." *CIBA Symposium.* Rpt., 12, (1964).

_____. "Traditional Therapies of Ancient India." *Sandoz News.* Rpt., 3, (1966).

Olschak, Blanche Christine in collaboration with Geshe Thupten Wangyal, *The Mystic Art of Ancient Tibet,* English translation © 1963 by George Allen and Unwin Ltd., published by McGraw-Hill Book Company, New York. ISBN 07-047523-7.

Patrul Rinpoche. *The Collected Works of dPal-sprul O-rgyan 'Jigs-med Chos-kyi dBang-po.* Gangtok, Sikkim: Sonam Topgay Kazi, 1970. Vol. 2.

Rechung Rinpoche, Jampal Kunzang. *Tibetan Medicine.* Berkeley: Univ. of California Press, 1973.

Samdhong Rinpoche. "Medical Therapy in Buddhism—Its Aim and Nature." *Religion and Medicine.* Ed. K. N. Udupa and G. Singh. Varanasi, India: Institute of Medical Sciences, BHU, 1974.

Shantideva. *A Guide to the Bodhisattva's Way of Life.* Trans. Stephen Batchelor. Dharamsala: Library of Tibetan Works and Archives, 1979.

Sigerist, Henry. *History of Medicine.* New York: Oxford Univ. Press, 1961. Vol. II.

Snellgrove, David and Hugh Richardson. *A Cultural History of Tibet.* New York: Frederick A. Praeger, 1968.

Stablein, William. "Tibetan Medical-Cultural System." *An Introduction to Tibetan Medicine.* Ed. Dawa Norbu. Delhi: Tibetan Review Publications, 1976.

Stcherbatsky, T. *The Central Conception of Buddhism: The Meaning of the Word Dharma.* 1923; rpt. Varanasi, India: Motilal Banarsidass, 1970.

Thoreau, Henry David, trans. "The White Lotus of the Good Law." *The Dial,* Vol. IV, (3), 1844.

Trungpa, Chogyam. *Cutting Through Spiritual Materialism.* Berkeley: Shambhala, 1973.

Tucci, Giuseppe. *The Theory and Practice of the Mandala.* Trans. A. H. Brodrick. 1969; rpt. New York: Samuel Weiser, 1973.

Udupa, K. N. and G. Singh. *Religion and Medicine.* Varanasi, India: Institute of Medical Sciences, Benares Hindu University, 1974.

Uphof, J. C. T. *Dictionary of Economic Plants.* 2nd ed. Lehre, Germany: Verlag Von J. Cramer, 1968.

Vogel, Claus. "On Bu-ston's View of the Eight Parts of Indian Medicine." *Indo-Iranian Journal,* 6, (1963), 290-5.

Waddell, L. A. *Tibetan Buddhism.* 1895; rpt. New York: Dover, 1972.

Wade, Carlson, *Health Secrets of the Orient.* West Nyack, N.Y.: Parker Publishing Co., 1973.

Wangyal, Geshe. *The Door of Liberation.* New York: Girodias, 1973.

Wayman, Alex. "Buddhist Tantric Medicine Theory." *An Introduction to Tibetan Medicine.* Ed. Dawa Norbu. Delhi: Tibetan Review Publications, 1976.

Willis, Janice D. *The Diamond Light of the Eastern Dawn.* New York: Simon & Schuster, 1971.

Zilboorg, Gregory. *A History of Medical Psychiatry.* New York: W. W. Norton & Co., (1941), 1967.

Zimmer, Heinrich. *Hindu Medicine.* Baltimore: The Johns Hopkins Press, 1948.

———. *Philosophies of India.* Ed. Joseph Campbell. Bollingen Series XXVI. New York: Meridian, 1951.

Typescripts, Unpublished Manuscripts, Transcripts, and Tape Recordings

Barshi Phuntsel Wangyal. "A Short Explanation of Tibetan Medicine." Trans. Lobsang Lhalungpa. Long Island: Bodhi House, 1976. Unpublished manuscript.

Chagmed Rinpoche. "Hymn in Praise of the Medicine Buddha." Trans. Sister Palmo and Trangu Rinpoche. Typescript. Seattle: Karma Rigdrol Publications, 1974.

Chandra, Lokesh. *A Sanskrit-Tibetan Dictionary of Medical Terms.* New Delhi: International Academy of Indian Culture. Unpublished manuscript.

Dhonden, Dr. Yeshi. "A Talk on Tibetan Humoral Medicine." New York: Dharmadhatu, 1974.

Doboom Rinpoche. "A Talk on Methods of Exorcism." Transcript. Dharamsala, 1976.

Dodrag Amchi Rinpoche. "Complete Teachings on Chapters 77, 78, and 79 of the *Man-Ngag-rGyud,* the Third Tantra of the *rGyud-bzhi.*" Kathmandu: Kedrup Sherab Ling Monastery, 1976. (Tapes.)

Dudjom Rinpoche, H. H. "Seminar on the Six Bardos." Transcript. Greenville, New York, 1980.

_____. "Seminar on Mind and Healing." New York: Yeshe Nyingpo, 1980 (Tapes.)

_____. "Talks on the Nature of Mind." New York, 1976.

_____. *Nyingma History.* Trans. Gyurmed Dorje and Matthew Kapstein. Unpublished manuscript.

Lobsang, Dr. Ama. "A Talk on Tibetan Psychiatry." Dharamsala, 1976. (Tapes.)

Pema Dorje. "Notes from a Class on Tibetan Medicine." Dharamsala, 1976. Transcript.

_____. "A Talk on Tibetan Psychiatry." Dharamsala, 1976. (Tapes.)

Romero, Philip. "Tibetan Medicine: An Ancient System Struggles to Survive." Unpublished manuscript.

Sogyal Rinpoche. "A Lecture on the Tibetan Art of Healing." London, 1975. Transcript.

Thinley Norbu Rinpoche. "Seminar on Tantric Practices according to the Nyingmapa Tradition." Transcript. New York: Yeshe Nyingpo, 1977.

Tulku Thondup Rinpoche. "A Summary of Mipham Rinpoche's Commentary on the Seven Line Prayer." Transcript. Providence: Mahasiddha Nyingmapa Center, 1977.

Wangla, Amchi Lama. "Teachings on the Medicine called 'The Precious Essence which Removes the Mind of Sorrow.'" Transcript. Ghoom, Darjeeling, 1976.

Yeshe Dorje Rinpoche. "Talks on Nagas, Exorcism, and Compassion." Dharamsala, 1976. (Tapes.)

Index